ON-CALL
in
Urology

Mr Hamid Abboudi
Consultant Urological Surgeon,
Imperial Urology, Imperial College Healthcare NHS Trust, UK

Miss Charlotte Dunford
Consultant Urological Surgeon,
Norfolk and Norwich NHS Foundation Trust, UK

Mr Andrew Chetwood
Consultant Urological Surgeon,
Frimley Health NHS Foundation Trust, UK

Foreword by:
Roland Morley
(immediate past-chair SAC urology)

Series editors:
Mr Karl F.B. Payne
Clinical Lecturer in Oral & Maxillofacial Surgery, University of Birmingham
Specialty Trainee in Oral and Maxillofacial Surgery, West Midlands Deanery

Mr Arpan S. Tahim
Specialty Trainee in Oral and Maxillofacial Surgery, London Deanery

Mr Alexander M.C. Goodson
Oral and Maxillofacial Surgery Consultant, Queen Alexandra Hospital, Portsmouth

First published in 2022 by Libri Publishing

ISBN 978-1-911450-65-8

A CIP catalogue record for this book is available from The British Library

Cover and Design by Carnegie Publishing

Printed in the UK by Halstan

Libri Publishing
Brunel House
Volunteer Way
Faringdon
Oxfordshire
SN7 7YR

Tel: +44 (0)845 873 3837

www.libripublishing.co.uk

CONTENTS

About the editorial team   vi

About the "On-call" series   vii

Dedication   viii

Acknowledgements   ix

Abbreviations   x

Foreword   xii

Introduction   1

Disclaimer   2

Chapter 1: Essentials   **3**

    1.1   Basics   3

    1.2   Referrals   4

    1.3   Admission clerking for elective patients   6

    1.4   Admission clerking for emergency patients   8

    1.5   Anatomy   10

    1.6   Radiology   11

    1.7   Drugs   13

    1.8   Instruments in urology   16

Chapter 2: The emergency department   **25**

    2.1   Renal colic   26

    2.2   The acute scrotum   28

    2.3   Haematuria   30

    2.4   Urinary tract infection and sepsis   31

    2.5   Urinary retention (including post-obstructive diuresis)   32

    2.6   Difficult catheterisation   34

    2.7   Paraphimosis   36

    2.8   Urological trauma   37

    2.9   Priapism   40

    2.10   Urological issues in pregnancy   42

2.11   Assessing a post-operative patient for ureteric injury   44

2.12   Paediatrics   45

Chapter 3: The ward   **47**

3.1   The ward round   47

3.2   Prescribing intravenous fluids   48

3.3   Post-obstructive diuresis   50

3.4   Patients with abnormal blood glucose   51

3.5   Anticoagulation   54

3.6   Nephrostomies and abdominal drains   55

3.7   Catheters and irrigation   56

3.8   Evaluating the acutely "unwell" patient   57

3.9   Common post-operative problems   59

Chapter 4: The clinic   **63**

4.1   Follow-up of acute ureteric colic   64

4.2   Scrotal swellings   65

4.3   Haematuria   67

4.4   Raised PSA   68

4.5   Male lower urinary tract symptoms   69

Chapter 5: The operating theatre   **71**

5.1   Classification of emergency surgery   71

5.2   The WHO surgical safety checklist   73

5.3   Placing a patient on the emergency list   74

5.4   Consent and marking   75

5.5   Preparing a patient for theatre   76

5.6   Benefits and risks of specific surgical procedures   77

5.6.1   Flexible cystoscopy   77

5.6.2   Rigid cystoscopy +/- bladder biopsy   77

5.6.3   Circumcision   78

5.6.4   Hydrocele repair   78

5.6.5   Scrotal exploration for suspected testicular torsion   79

5.6.6   Ureteric stent insertion   80

5.6.7   Suprapubic catheter insertion   80

5.7   What to ask your scrub nurse for   81

Chapter 6: Practical procedures   **83**

6.1   Venepuncture, IV cannulation, taking blood cultures

          and arterial blood gases   83

6.2   Urine analysis – dipsticks, MSU, CSU, βHCG   88

6.3   Urethral catheterisation   91

6.4   Suprapubic catheterisation   93

6.5   Penile block   95

6.6   Reduction of a paraphimosis   96

Author biographies   **97**

Index   **99**

ABOUT THE EDITORIAL TEAM

Mr Karl F.B. Payne

BMedSci (Hons) BMBS BDS MRCS PhD

Clinical Lecturer in Oral & Maxillofacial Surgery, University of Birmingham

Specialty Trainee in Oral and Maxillofacial Surgery, West Midlands Deanery

Mr Arpan S. Tahim

BSc (Hons) MBBS BDS MRCS MEd PhD

Specialty Trainee in Oral and Maxillofacial Surgery, London Deanery

Mr Alexander M.C. Goodson

BSc (Hons) FRCS (OMFS) DOHNS

Oral and Maxillofacial Surgery Consultant, Queen Alexandra Hospital, Portsmouth

ABOUT THE ON-CALL SERIES

The "On-call" series is a unique learning resource consisting of concise, accessible and highly readable books. Authored and edited by a team with a strong focus on medical and surgical education, they have proven to be highly useful both for junior doctors seeking guidance early on in their clinical rotations and for those with more experience who are looking to consolidate and develop their knowledge. Written as "survival guides," each book covers common presentations in the emergency, ward and clinic settings, along with detailed step-by-step descriptions of typical surgical procedures. The attention to hands-on practical advice with easy-to-follow instructions means they are the only handbooks that a junior trainee should not be without.

DEDICATION

The authors would like to dedicate this book to their respective families. We thank them for their patience, understanding and limitless support in our professional endeavours.

Mr Hamid Abboudi BSc (Hons), MBBS, PG CERT HBE, FRCS (Urol)

Consultant Urological Surgeon, Imperial Urology, Imperial College Healthcare NHS Trust, UK

Miss Charlotte Dunford MBBS, BSc (Hons), FRCS (Urol)

Consultant Urological Surgeon, Norfolk and Norwich NHS Foundation Trust, UK

Mr Andrew Chetwood BMedSci (Hons), MBChB (Hons), FRCS (Urol)

Consultant Urological Surgeon, Frimley Health NHS Foundation Trust, UK

ACKNOWLEDGEMENTS

We would like to thank Dr Giuseppe Celentano, Consultant Urological Surgeon, Department of Neurosciences, Sciences of Reproduction, and Odontostomatology, University of Naples Federico II, Naples, Italy, for his contribution towards the images.

ABBREVIATIONS

ABG	arterial blood gas
AFP	alpha fetoprotein
ATLS	advanced trauma life support
AUR	acute urinary retention
BAUS	British Association of Urological Surgeons
bd	twice a day
βHCG	beta human chorionic gonadotropin
CT KUB	computed tomography of kidneys, ureters and bladder (non-contrast)
CTPA	computed tomography pulmonary angiogram
CTU	Computer tomography scan of abdomen and pelvis with urographic phases (delayed)
DEXA	dual-energy X-ray absorptiometry
DKA	diabetic ketoacidosis
DMSA scan	dimercaptosuccinic acid scan
DRE	digital rectal examination
ECG	electrocardiogram
ED	emergency department
FBC	full blood count
FY1	foundation year 1 doctor
FY2	foundation year 2 doctor
G&S	group and save
Hb	haemoglobin
HHS	hyperosmolar hyperglycaemic state
HoLEP	holmium laser enucleation of the prostate
IM	intramuscular
INR	international normalised ratio
ITU	intensive therapy unit
IV	intravenous
JVP	jugular venous pressure
kg	kilogram(s)
L	litre(s)
LDH	lactate dehydrogenase
LMWH	low molecular weight heparin
MAG3 scan	mercaptoacetyltriglycine scan
MDT	Multidisciplinary team
mg	milligram(s)
ml	millilitre(s)

mmol	millimole(s)
MRI	magnetic resonance imaging
MRSA	methicillin-resistant *Staphylococcus aureus*
MSU	mid-stream urine (sample)
mSv	millisievert
NBM	nil by mouth
NCEPOD	National Confidential Enquiry into Patient Outcome and Death
NOAC	novel oral anticoagulant
NSAID	non-steroidal anti-inflammatory drug
PCNL	percutaneous nephrolithotomy
PO	per oral route of administration
POC	package of care
PPI	proton pump inhibitor (e.g. omeprazole)
PR	per rectum
PSA	prostate specific antigen
qds	four times a day
SC	subcutaneous
SPC	suprapubic catheter
SpR	specialist registrar
tds	three times a day
TEDS	thrombo-embolic deterrent stockings
TURP	transurethral resection of prostate
TWOC	trial without catheter
U&E	urea and electrolytes (serum creatinine included)
US	ultrasound scan
US KUB	ultrasound of kidneys, ureters and bladder
UTI	urinary tract infection
VE	vaginal examination
VTE	venous thromboembolism
WCC	white cell count

FOREWORD

Urology is an interesting and challenging speciality covering many aspects of medical and surgical care in patients of all ages. Exposure to urology before qualifying is very limited and yet up to 25% of emergency surgery contains elements of urology. *On-call in Urology* provides a simple and concise approach for managing common emergency and elective urological problems. This book will put the reader at ease and I have no hesitation in recommending this book to junior doctors to help them learn quickly.

Roland Morley (immediate past-chair SAC urology)

INTRODUCTION

Urology relates to the surgical and medical management of urinary tract disease. It is a fantastic surgical speciality primarily because it engages all patients regardless of age or assigned gender, and has a breadth of pathology reaching from benign to malignant disease. As a urologist you will manage both men and women, young and old. Urological training comprises extensive general urological exposure with sub-specialisation including oncology, female, paediatric, reconstruction, andrology, stones and functional aspects.

We are very involved in all aspects of our patients' care pathway, performing much of our own diagnostics, and have often been at the forefront of innovation in surgical technique. Exposure to urology is often not extensive in medical school and for this reason many newly qualified doctors can find it a little daunting. We have written this book as a practical guide to navigating life as a junior doctor in urology. We hope you find it full of useful tips to make your time working in urology enjoyable and even consider it as a career in the future!

DISCLAIMER

This book is not a textbook, but a survival guide. All the content has been written by the authors and is obtained from reliable sources and based on personal experience. The authors have no affiliations or conflicts of interest to declare regarding this book. The authors and publisher do not accept responsibility or legal liability for injury or damage to any person as a result of action or refraining from action due to the clinical material within this book. At the time of printing, drug doses contained within the book were correct, but it is the reader's responsibility to check up-to-date manufacturer and drug dose safety guidelines.

CHAPTER 1: ESSENTIALS

1.1 BASICS

Urology, like many surgical specialities, is logical and based on key principles. Likened to "plumbing", the first thing to remember is that the urinary system flows from the top (kidneys) to the bottom (urethra). Normally there is no pressure in the system, as a compliant bladder expands to fill with urine and keep pressures low. Any blockage in outflow, wherever it is along the urinary tract, will cause problems upstream of where the obstruction is. The objective in an *emergency* setting is to relieve that obstruction and create a low-pressure urinary system, draining safely. In principle, this is facilitated using catheters, stents or nephrostomies.

As a rule of thumb, before starting any urology job, make sure you know which senior is supporting you and how you can get hold of them. Familiarise yourself with the department and where you can find equipment you will need (e.g. catheters, guidewires). Learn from the experienced nursing staff in the department, who will be more than happy to teach you their tips and tricks for getting out of bother. Be organised in your thoughts and approach to patient care. Keep your management plans simple and easy to implement, and above all, make sure the patient is at the centre of all your management decisions. Know your limitations and always ask for help when you need it.

1.2 REFERRALS

ESSENTIALS

MAKING REFERRALS

When making a referral it is important to put yourself in the receiving person's shoes. What information would you want to know? Remember they are busy too, so it is essential to be clear and concise in what you are asking for.

Firstly, make sure you are contacting the correct person. Different hospitals have different referral systems and some are now moving towards specialities having on-call phones as opposed to bleeps/pagers. Generally speaking, medical teams prefer you to refer to the on-call senior doctor, and may have a different senior responsible for ward problems and another for emergency admissions. In most surgical specialities, the on-call junior surgical doctor takes the referral, but check this in your own hospital.

Secondly, ensure you have the correct patient details, including a name, hospital number, date of birth and location. It is useful to pre-empt and prepare yourself for possible questions they might ask – for example, about blood and imaging results. It is always polite to start by introducing yourself, stating your name and grade. Next, it is best to state your intentions – for example, "can I refer a patient to you, please?" rather than "can I ask your advice, please?" will make it clear to whoever you are speaking with exactly what you are asking them for. Explain why the patient was admitted to hospital (keep this succinct and relevant) and their past medical history, then get on to why you want them to see the patient. They may ask you to arrange investigations and give you instructions on how to manage the patient while they are waiting to be seen. It is important to document these conversations and instructions in the notes, with a time, date and who you spoke to (name and grade).

> **TOP TIP:**
>
> 1. Prepare: have the patient's details, past medical history, drug history and latest investigation results to hand
>
> 2. Be polite: introduce yourself and state your grade
>
> 3. State your intention – for example, referral or advice
>
> 4. Be succinct: presenting complaint, relevant background and past medical history
>
> 5. Explain why you want them to see the patient
>
> 6. Document in the notes: date, time, name and grade of person you spoke to

ESSENTIALS

If you are not sure of any of these points, it is advisable to consult with a senior colleague before making the referral.

HOW TO RECEIVE REFERRALS

Urology is often viewed as a super-specialised area by other medical teams, such that whilst it is extremely common for patients (e.g. reduced mobility, on anticoagulants, diabetic, etc.) to have urological problems, many doctors do not feel confident dealing with issues that can arise. As a consequence, you will find that you are contacted about a variety of problems ranging from blocked or dislodged catheters to major trauma. We will now go through the important things you need to consider when accepting a referral, the salient questions to ask and the investigations to request prior to your review.

It is important to ascertain the following things: name and age of the patient, where the patient is, what relevant medical problems they have (e.g. reduced mobility, on anticoagulants, diabetic with sepsis, etc.), what issue the referring team wants help with and what question they want answering. Often you will be asked about non-urgent management plans or to help arrange outpatient investigations. If you are not sure, remember to ask the referrer for their name and contact details, and explain you will get back to them as soon as you have discussed it with your senior.

1.3 ADMISSION CLERKING FOR ELECTIVE PATIENTS

Most hospitals have a nurse-led pre-assessment department but it is very important that you are aware of two essential components to admitting a patient for elective surgery. Ensure, firstly, that the patient still requires the operation and, secondly, that they are medically fit for an anaesthetic and the surgery proposed. Most hospital trusts will have clerking proformas which you should fill out. In their absence, there are a few essentials you must document:

1. Your name, grade, date and time of clerking
2. Patient details – age and sex
3. Reason for hospital attendance, e.g. elective admission for laparoscopic radical nephrectomy
4. Past medical history (including any recent illness, e.g. chest infection)
5. Drug history and drug allergies (including latex – important to know as these patients must be first on the operating list for the day)
6. Social history: particularly important in elderly patients (include package of care details)
7. VTE assessment (including prescribing thrombo-prophylaxis on the drug chart)
8. Examine the patient (all major systems) and check a urine dip
9. Ensure the patient is NBM for the correct period of time (at least 6 hours for food, 2 hours for clear fluids)
10. Check pre-operative assessment results: patient MRSA status, blood and MSU results (ensure patients haven't arrived with untreated anaemia or UTIs).

Routine bloods, mid-stream urine sample (MSU) and methicillin-resistant *Staphylococcus aureus* (MRSA) swabs should have already been taken at pre-operative assessment. You should personally check all these results to ensure patients haven't arrived with untreated anaemia or a urinary tract infection (UTI). Furthermore, for certain cases, patients will need a valid group-and-save (G&S) sample in case a blood transfusion is later required. Your hospital will have its own protocol for which operations require these and a list should be available in your department. However, a summary of common urological procedures warranting pre-operative G&S is listed in Table 1.1. If in doubt, send a G&S sample.

ESSENTIALS

Common urological procedures requiring a valid pre-op G&S
Cystectomy/cystoprostatectomy (open/laparoscopic/robotic)
Nephrectomy/partial nephrectomy (open/laparoscopic/robotic)
Prostatectomy (open/laparoscopic/robotic)
Percutaneous nephrolithotomy (PCNL)
Transurethral resection of prostate (TURP)/bladder tumour (TURBT) or laser prostatectomy (e.g. HOLEP)*

These operations have a very low transfusion rate so please check your local policy and/or speak with the operating surgeon.

Table 1.1: Blood transfusion requirements

Patients over the age of 50 years should also have a routine ECG at pre-operative assessment. Ensure the results are present in the notes before the surgeon or anaesthetist sees them, to help avoid unnecessary delays (the admitting nursing staff will often help you with this).

TOP TIP:

Most patients will have had all the relevant imaging they need prior to the operation and this will have been checked by the surgeon in clinic or through the MDT. Sometimes however, particularly when patients are listed very quickly for operations, the pre-operative imaging may not have always been checked. An example is those patients with suspected testicular tumours scheduled for a radical orchidectomy. These patients must have a CXR (to look for pulmonary metastasis before an anaesthetic) and it is worth checking they have had one and, if not, arranging it to avoid delay.

The next step is to consent and mark the patient. Consent should be taken by someone who understands the risks, benefits and alternatives to a procedure as well as being competent in performing the procedure. Therefore, unless you are happy that you fit all these criteria, please consult with your senior beforehand. Further details about consent are given in Chapter 5.

1.4 ADMISSION CLERKING FOR EMERGENCY PATIENTS

The format for clerking in emergency patients is very similar, and in most hospitals, you would use the same clerking proforma. You will need to take a focused urological history from the patient, which may be based around the following:

1. Your name, grade, date and time of clerking
2. Patient details: age and sex
3. Presenting complaint, e.g. acute urinary retention
4. Past medical history (and relevant urological history)
5. Drug history and drug allergies
6. Social history: particularly important in elderly patients (include package of care details)
7. VTE assessment and prescription of thrombo-prophylaxis on the drug chart
8. Examine the patient (+/- DRE), including baseline observations (temperature, heart rate, etc.)
9. Decide if the patient needs to be NBM and document this.

Having taken a focussed history, review any previous clinic letters, arrange essential investigations such as imaging (Table 1.2) and blood tests (Table 1.3), and check microbiology results, before formulating a differential diagnosis and your subsequent management plan.

Presentation	Required investigations
Renal colic	urine dip, βHCG (if applicable), MSU, CT KUB and bloods (U&E, serum calcium and uric acid)
Acute urinary retention	urine dip, MSU, bloods-U&E (and US KUB if creatinine abnormal) and **importantly, document the residual volume on catheterisation!**
Visible haematuria	urine dip, MSU and bloods (Hb and U&E), CT urogram/US KUB (depending on a patient's comorbidity and performance status)
Acute testicular pain	urine dip

Table 1.2: Essential investigations

Important urological blood tests
Serum creatinine, urea and electrolytes (U&E)
Full blood count (FBC)
Prostate specific antigen (PSA)
Clotting function (coagulation screen) +/- INR
Serum calcium and urate/uric acid

Table 1.3: Essential blood tests

It is sensible to discuss all patients you see with a senior when starting out in your urology career. If you are confident of your diagnoses and management plans, it may be sufficient to do this as a "paper round" at the end of the day. Otherwise, if you are unsure, or the patient is unwell, you should discuss each case with your senior as you admit them. More detail on how to manage each urological emergency will be discussed later in the book.

ESSENTIALS

1.5 ANATOMY

The anatomy comprises the kidneys, ureters, bladder and urethra, with the addition of penis and scrotum in males (figures 1.1 and 1.2).

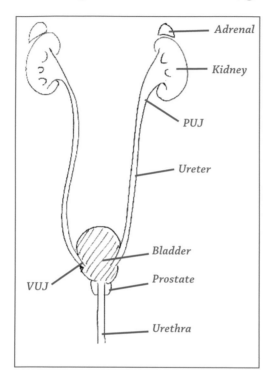

Figure 1.1: Schematic anatomy of the urinary tract

Figure 1.2: Pelvic anatomy with areas of the genito-urinary tract highlighted: bladder/urethra (GREEN); prostate (PURPLE); epididymis, vas deferens, seminal vesicle and ejaculatory duct (ORANGE); testes (YELLOW); corpora spongiosum (BLUE); corpora cavernosa (GREY)

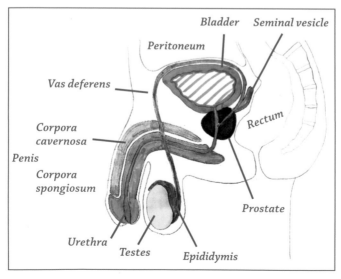

1.6 RADIOLOGY

A close understanding of radiology is integral to being a urologist. Below is a brief description of the common scans you will request, including their radiation dose.

Plain X-ray KUB (0.6mSv) – As a comparison, a CXR is 0.02mSv and the annual background radiation dose in the UK is 2–3mSv. 50–60% of stones are visible on plain film and plain films still have a role in the outpatient management of stone disease.

X-ray screening in theatre (variable dose) is often needed for ureteroscopic and renal stone surgery (URS/PCNL), stent insertion and on-table cystogram. It usually requires booking in advance, so you should check whether you require it at the earliest opportunity.

Intravenous urogram (IVU) (1.5mSv) – In most situations, this has been superseded by CT urography. It requires the administration of a tri-iodinated contrast media with subsequent delayed films taken to depict filling of the collecting system. It still has a role in some units for the assessment of ureteric colic and is also used in an on-table IVU in renal trauma and in some post-op scenarios. If using IV contrast, it is important to be aware of the complications that can arise (allergy, renal impairment and anaphylaxis) and how to manage them.

Urethrogram (variable dose) – This has a role in the emergency assessment of urethral trauma and assessment of urethral stricture disease. A hysteroscopy catheter (which has a small balloon) can be inserted into the fossa navicularis so antegrade and retrograde images can be taken as the contrast medium is injected and then voided.

Cystogram (variable dose) – This is the administration of contrast via a urethral catheter. It is used to ensure the bladder has healed after trauma or when the bladder has been opened and then repaired in a planned fashion. The usual protocol is to take a control film and then administer 50ml of contrast to assess for a large leak. Then a total of 150–300ml is instilled looking for a smaller leak. Finally, a post-drainage film is taken, including at an oblique view to identify a posterior leak.

ESSENTIALS

Ultrasound (no dose) – This is a radiation-free modality which uses a piezo-electric crystal to produce high-frequency ultrasound waves. This is used in abdominal imaging (US KUB) to assess for hydronephrosis, renal masses/stones, ureteric dilation/calculi (in proximal or distal ureter) and post-void bladder residuals. US provides excellent images of the testes. Doppler or colour duplex can be deployed to assess for flow characteristics.

CT (variable up to 15mSv) uses X-rays produced and detected on a rotating gantry to develop a 3D cross-sectional image of the body. Non-contrast CT KUB is the gold standard in initial investigation of suspected ureteric colic and has a high sensitivity and specificity. Its radiation dose is 1–5mSv although modern low dose scanners can be less than 1mSv. Intravenous contrast can be administered for a contrast CT scan. A CT renal utilises an arterial, parenchymal and portal-venous phase to assess for renal masses and enhancement. A CT urogram utilises a delayed excretory phase to allow the collecting system to fill with contrast. A CT urogram may be up to 15mSv.

MRI (no dose) exploits the spin characteristics of hydrogen atoms in water molecules. Using pulses of energy to manipulate the magnetic field applied to the hydrogen atoms results in energy release, which is amplified to give the MR signal. MRI is used for assessment/diagnosis of prostate cancer, staging of prostate cancer, assessment of the indeterminate renal mass, staging in bladder cancer and can be used for the staging of penile cancer.

Nuclear medicine scans include MAG3 and DMSA scans, which give an idea of renal function and drainage. A DMSA scan gives a detailed assessment of split renal function. A MAG3 renogram also provides information on drainage of each kidney and is useful when assessing for obstruction. A DEXA scan is used to assess bone density.

1.7 DRUGS

ANALGESICS

When prescribing analgesics for pain you should adhere to the World Health Organization "pain ladder". This describes a stepwise approach, starting with weaker analgesics and moving through the different strength opioids.

1) Non-opioid

Paracetamol 1g PO/IV qds +/- non-steroidal anti-inflammatory drug (NSAID)

Diclofenac 75–150mg PR daily in divided doses

Ibuprofen 400mg PO tds, max. 2.4g daily

N.B. Use NSAIDs with extreme caution in patients with renal or hepatic impairment, or a history of cardiovascular disease. Consult the medical team if in doubt.

2) Weak opioid

Codeine phosphate 30–60mg PO/IM 4 hourly, max. 240mg daily

Dihydrocodeine 30mg PO 4–6 hourly

Tramadol 50–100mg PO/IM/IV 4 hourly, max. 400 mg daily

3) Strong opioid

Morphine sulphate oral liquid (Oramorph) 5–10mg 4 hourly

Morphine SC/IV 5–10mg 4 hourly

Oxynorm (oral oxycodone) 5mg PO 4–6 hourly, titrate as necessary, max. 400mg daily

Oxycodone 1–10mg IV 4 hourly

When using morphine to manage acute pain it is acceptable to titrate up the dose by 5–10mg every 30 minutes to achieve adequate pain control. Be aware of the risk of opiate overdose, its symptoms and acute management. Use an initial dose of 2.5–5mg in frail or elderly patients. Your hospital will likely have approved pain guidelines to refer to and the above should be used as guidance only.

ESSENTIALS

ANTI-EMETICS

Post-operative nausea and vomiting are common. Prescribing an anti-emetic, as required, for all patients is recommended. It is important to note that each anti-emetic has a specific mode of action, as detailed in the table below. Therefore, escalating one drug to a similar mode of drug is unlikely to alleviate the symptoms of the patient. A combination of anti-emetics with different modes of action will be more effective.

Drug	Dose	Mechanism of action
Cyclizine	PO/IM/IV 500mg tds	Antihistamine
Prochlorperazine	PO 20mg initially, then 10mg 2 hourly; IM 12.5mg qds	Antidopaminergic
Ondansetron	PO/IM/IV 4mg tds	$5HT_3$ receptor antagonist
Domperidone	PO 10–20mg tds	Antidopaminergic/prokinetic
Metoclopramide	PO/IM/IV 10mg tds	Prokinetic

Table 1.4: Anti-emetic drugs

ANTIBIOTICS

When prescribing antibiotics empirically, you must follow your local microbiology department guidance as this will be based on the resistance pattern of pathogens in the local community of patients you treat. It is essential that you check your local hospital antibiotic policy to avoid empirically prescribing an antibiotic which has wide resistance in your area. It is better still to prescribe an antibiotic based on previous culture and sensitivities of any prior infections. The antibiotics listed below are not an exhaustive list, but should be the main agents you will encounter. Your hospital's antibiotic guidelines should also detail specific dose regiments for each infection (as these can vary between hospitals also). Advice should be sought from the microbiology department if in doubt.

Drug	Dose
Amoxicillin	PO 250–500mg bd
	IM/IV 500mg tds; IV 1g qds in severe infection
Co-amoxiclav	PO 625mg tds
	IV 1.2g tds
Cefuroxime	PO 250–500 mg bd
	IM/IV 750mg–1.5g tds (depending on severity of infection)
Gentamicin	IV 3–5mg per kg stat dose; for once-daily dose regimen, consult local guidelines on monitoring serum gentamicin concentration
Metronidazole	PO 200–500mg qds
	IV 500mg tds
Nitrofurantoin	PO 50mg qds
Trimethoprim	PO 200mg bd

Table 1.5: Antibiotics

ESSENTIALS

1.8 INSTRUMENTS IN UROLOGY

In this section we will discuss the essential urological instruments you need to know about, and those that you might come across whilst on-call. There are of course many more advanced instruments to be aware of should you pursue a career in urology in the future.

URETHRAL CATHETERS

Two-way urethral catheters are so named because they have two channels: one to drain urine and a separate channel filled with sterile water to inflate the balloon and hold the catheter in place. This channel usually has a coloured toggle on it and the connecting end fits a normal syringe tip (not a Luer lock syringe). The coloured toggles are different, depending on the size of the catheter. Gauges and their colour coding can vary between manufacturers, however. Table 1.6 illustrates the common colour coding of catheter sizes.

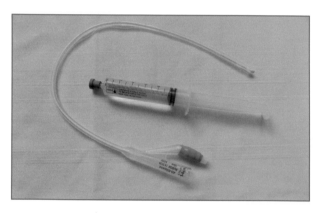

Figure 1.3: 2-way catheter

Catheter size	Toggle colour	Potential use
12Ch 2-way	White	Female patients
14Ch 2-way	Green	Female or male patients
16Ch 2-way	Orange	Male patients in AUR
18Ch 2-way	Red	Male patients in AUR
20Ch 3-way	White	Female/male patients with visible haematuria
22Ch 3-way	Purple	Female/male patients with visible haematuria

Table 1.6: Catheter guide

ESSENTIALS

Most 2-way catheters are packaged with a pre-filled syringe containing 10ml of sterile water to fill the catheter balloon with. There are of course some exceptions and therefore you should always check the catheter packaging, where the intended volume for the balloon will be displayed. Then you will need to locate a syringe and draw up that volume of sterile water yourself.

> **TOP TIP:**
>
> Some hospital trusts will stock female and male catheter lengths: female catheters are shorter in length and many hospitals have stopped stocking them. This is as a result of incidents where female catheters were inserted into male patients and the balloon is inflated in the prostatic urethra, despite being inserted to the hilt, resulting in traumatic catheterisation. Check within your trust if female catheters are available and always check the catheter you have is appropriate for your patient before using it.

ESSENTIALS

Three-way urethral catheters have a third channel, which allows irrigation to flow continuously through it. You should note which channel is for irrigation and which is for attaching the catheter bag to. Attach the catheter bag to the larger middle channel and the irrigation tubing to the smaller channel to the side. (Again, the coloured toggle marks the balloon port.) It is important that you get this correct. If you attach the irrigation to the catheter draining channel, you will fill the bladder very quickly. Conversely, the catheter will not drain well out of the irrigation channel. The consequence is that the bladder will overfill and you will make the patient incredibly uncomfortable and risk perforating the bladder.

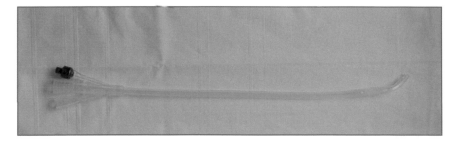

Figure 1.4: 3-way catheter

SUPRAPUBIC CATHETERS (SPCS)

These are no different to a 2-way catheter. Therefore, if you are changing one for a patient with an existing SPC, simply select a 2-way urethral catheter of the corresponding size to do this. However, if you are inserting an SPC into a patient for the first time, you will need to find an SPC kit like the one shown in Figure 1.5. This kit uses the Seldinger principle for insertion and everything is available in this tray. The only thing you'll need to bring is a catheter bag and some local anaesthetic. Your hospital may have other SPC insertion kits which don't use this principle. Unless you are familiar with them, or being supervised by a senior who is familiar with them, it is often safer to use the Seldinger kits. How to put in an SPC is discussed in more detail later on in this book.

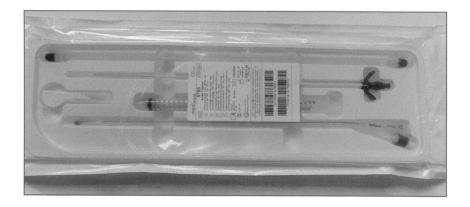

Figure 1.5: Suprapubic catheter kit

BLADDER SYRINGE

The bladder syringe has a pointed tapered end, which fits easily into the drainage channel of any catheter. This is required to perform a bladder washout.

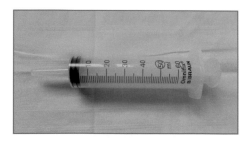

Figure 1.6: Bladder syringe

LOCAL ANAESTHETIC CONTAINING LUBRICATING GEL (E.G. INSTILLAGEL®)

Instillagel® is the trade name for a pre-filled syringe containing a lubricating gel with local anaesthetic and antiseptic solution. They come in 6ml and 11ml syringes, and 6ml is enough for female catheterisation. However, when catheterising a male patient, you will need a minimum of one 11ml tube. If the patient is known to have an enlarged prostate it is often sensible to squirt more than one tube of gel down the urethra before attempting catheterisation.

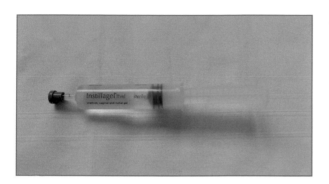

Figure 1.7: Instillagel®

CATHETER BAGS

Catheter bags come in several varieties for different purposes. Urometer bags hold at least two litres of urine and have a harder plastic box into which the catheter drains, initially allowing for hourly urine output measurement before it is discarded into the larger soft plastic bag behind it.

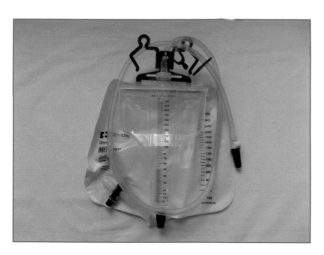

Figure 1.8: Urometer bag

ESSENTIALS

Leg bags hold 500ml and are designed so that Velcro straps can be threaded through them and secured to the patient's leg. They have an attachment at the top for the catheter, and a tap at the bottom to allow ease of emptying into the toilet.

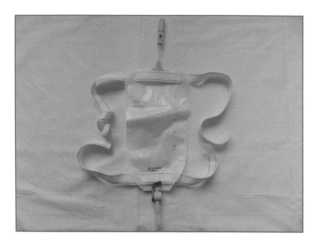

Figure 1.9: Leg bag

Night bags are standard soft plastic bags that hold two litres of urine. They are swapped over instead of a leg bag for use overnight, so that the patient can sleep through without having to wake to empty the smaller 500ml leg bag. They are also the most commonly seen catheter bag, particularly on medical wards. There are even larger soft catheter bags, which hold three litres. These are most commonly used for patients requiring irrigation, as the volume drained from the catheter is significantly more. This saves the nursing staff from having to repeatedly empty the bags.

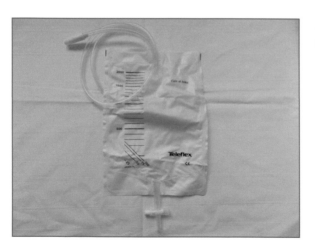

Figure 1.10: Standard night bags

FLEXIBLE CYSTOSCOPE

The flexible cystoscope is an instrument used to visualise the urethra, bladder outlet and bladder in the awake patient with the help of some local anaesthetic gel for lubrication. The flexibility of the instrument not only makes it more tolerable for the patient than a rigid instrument, but also allows a range of movement via the lever situated at the top of the scope, moved with your thumb. There is a channel to the front, which takes a normal "giving set" with a Luer lock attachment. You will need to run irrigation on inserting a scope, to open up the urethra and fill the bladder for inspection once you are in. The light lead is built into this instrument, usually within the camera connection, and this simply needs to be plugged into a video stack system to give you a picture on the monitor. Older flexible cystoscopes will have an eyepiece at the top, through which you can inspect the bladder lining, once you have connected the light lead to a source. Your department will run daily flexible cystoscopy lists and it is useful to learn how to use this instrument. If you are unable to catheterise a patient, direct vision afforded by the flexible cystoscope will help you navigate into the patient's bladder. You can then place a guidewire down the irrigation channel, leave this in the bladder, remove the scope and pass a catheter over this wire.

ESSENTIALS

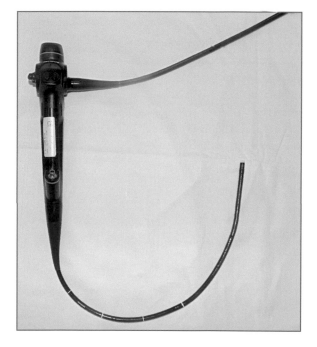

Figure 1.11: Flexible cystoscope

RIGID CYSTOSCOPE

The rigid cystoscope is used for a more formal inspection of the urethra, bladder outlet and bladder under general anaesthesia. It has a telescope with an attachment for the light source lead. The camera head is fixed onto the end of the telescope lens so that the image can be displayed on a monitor. Traditionally, the urologist looked through the end of the telescope directly. The telescope fits into a sheath which allows you to attach an irrigation supply to the side of it. With some lubricating gel, you are then ready to introduce the scope and inspect the patient's lower urinary tract.

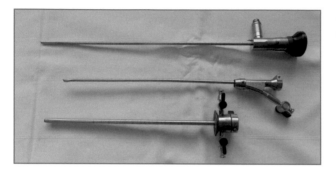

Figure 1.12: Rigid cystoscope

GUIDEWIRE

A guidewire is something you would use either to help you with a difficult catheterisation (as described above) or to help you place a stent into the ureter in order to relieve an obstruction. There are many different guidewires available and although you would have senior supervision when using any of these within the ureter, it is helpful to know the basics. Standard PTFE guidewires are the cheapest and most widely used. They are green, have one flexible end and one stiff end. It is important you make sure it is the flexible end that you introduce into the ureter.

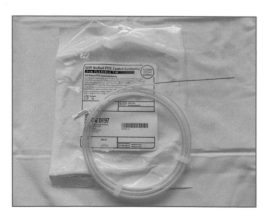

Figure 1.13: PTFE wire

The next most commonly used wire is a Sensor™ wire, which has a hydrophilic, very flexible black tip. The rest of the wire is blue. These are useful in oedematous ureters as they are less traumatic.

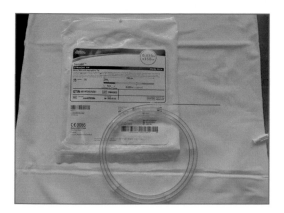

Figure 1.14: Sensor™ wire

URETERIC STENT

Ureteric stents, also known as "JJ stents" or "double J stents", are long, thin, plastic tubes of varying diameter designed to span the ureter and relieve an obstruction (e.g. ureteric calculi). They come in a variety of lengths and diameters. They have pigtail curls at either end, to anchor the stent in position in the renal pelvis and the bladder (hence the "double J"). They are inserted into the ureter with the aid of a rigid cystoscope, a guidewire and an image intensifier. You will need senior supervision when inserting a ureteric stent into an anaesthetised patient, but it is a core skill worth learning early on if you intend to pursue a career in urology.

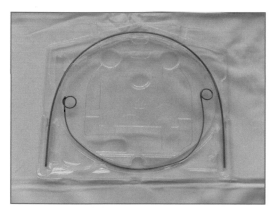

Figure 1.15: Ureteric stent

CHAPTER 2: THE EMERGENCY DEPARTMENT

Depending on local policies, acute urological presentations are seen either by a urology or a general surgical team member. It is important to see these patients promptly and to establish a diagnosis rapidly. In the following chapter, we describe the diagnosis and management of the common urological emergencies you may be asked to see in an emergency department (ED), in a surgical admissions unit (SAU) or on a ward.

2.1 RENAL COLIC

Renal (or ureteric) colic is the passage of a stone along the ureter. It is intensely painful and some female patients describe the pain as worse than childbirth. The history is of sudden-onset, severe pain originating in the loin, which can radiate to the groin or even genitals. The patient is unable to lie still, which can help in differentiation from peritonitis. The patient frequently feels nauseated and may describe some haematuria. Despite this "classical" history, only 50% of patients with such a history will have a proven stone on CT.

> **TOP TIP:**
>
> There are two key questions to ask when a patient is referred to you with a potential ureteric colic. *"Am I missing a potentially more serious diagnosis such as ruptured abdominal aortic aneurysm, perforated viscus, referred pain from myocardial infarction or ruptured ectopic pregnancy?"* Labelling a patient as having "renal colic" incorrectly can have dire consequences; if you have any concerns, you should communicate this with the referrer and/or your senior after you have assessed the patient. Some think that referral to urology with ureteric colic should only happen after the diagnosis is confirmed on a CT KUB. The second question is *"does the patient have an infected and obstructed kidney?"* This is a genuine urological emergency requiring prompt surgical decompression (ureteric stent or nephrostomy) with senior urology, radiology and sometimes ITU input

Key points in the history include a full pain history and past medical history, including previous stones and whether they required intervention. A history of anticoagulation, fever, and when the patient last ate and drank is important. The examination should include a full set of observations including temperature, examination of the abdomen to assess for an aortic aneurysm or peritonitis, urinalysis and blood tests (full blood count, urea and electrolytes, liver function tests, amylase and a clotting screen). Not all patients with ureteric colic will have haematuria (visible or non-visible). Female patients should have a urinary pregnancy test.

Most units now have access to prompt non-contrast CT KUB imaging. This is a highly sensitive and specific test and will confirm or exclude the presence of a stone. It also has the advantage of being able to identify other pathology and does not require intravenous contrast. Some units still utilise IVUs as a first-line investigation and you should be aware of local policies, and in particular the risks and management of anaphylaxis with using contrast.

Having established the diagnosis of ureteric colic, the next step is to rule out sepsis. A fever is the most sensitive marker of infection and most commonly a temperature greater than 38°C is regarded as significant. It is also important to check the contra-lateral kidney on the CT to ensure it is normal. An obstructed solitary kidney is another indication for intervention. Assuming there is no evidence of co-existing infection, the management of the stone within the ureter is based upon its size, how far it has left to travel through the urinary tract and how the patient has responded to analgesia. NSAIDs (e.g. Diclofenac 50–100mg PR) appear to be the most useful analgesic in managing colic as long as not contra-indicated. Acutely, patients can often require intravenous opiates and the addition of paracetamol maximises analgesic effects.

As a general rule, stones less than 5mm in size and in the distal ureter have a good chance of passage. A patient with a small stone and no evidence of infection who has their pain under control can be managed as an outpatient. The use of a plain X-ray KUB prior to discharge is not required if the scout film on the CT shows the stone; however, in some situations it can be useful. Traditionally, an alpha-blocker such as tamsulosin was prescribed to aid stone passage (medical expulsive therapy – MET) although a recent randomised controlled clinical trial failed to show any benefit in stone passage rates. As a general rule, as the urology on-call doctor, the key aim would be for you to decide if the patient needs admission or can be referred for outpatient management. This includes observation of small asymptomatic stones, lithotripsy, ureteroscopy and laser, and finally percutaneous stone surgery for larger renal stones.

EMERGENCY DEPARTMENT

2.2 THE ACUTE SCROTUM

The concern with acute scrotal pain is of torsion of the spermatic cord resulting in ischaemia to – and if untreated, necrosis of – the testis (Figure 2.1a). This should be your first diagnosis to exclude when referred a patient with acute scrotal pain. It is crucial to assess patients presenting with acute scrotal pain straight away. Ask about and clearly document the timeline of the symptoms. The longer the duration of pain, the less likely it is that testicular salvage is possible. The age of the patient is very important as torsion is unusual in pre-pubertal boys, and in this age group a torted hydatid of Morgagni (Figure 2.1b) or epididymitis is more likely to be the cause. Specifically ask about previous torsion, previous scrotal surgery, recent trauma and sexually transmitted infection. Remember that a small proportion of testicular tumours can present with pain and that non-scrotal conditions (e.g. ureteric colic, leaking abdominal aortic aneurysms) can also present with acute scrotal pain.

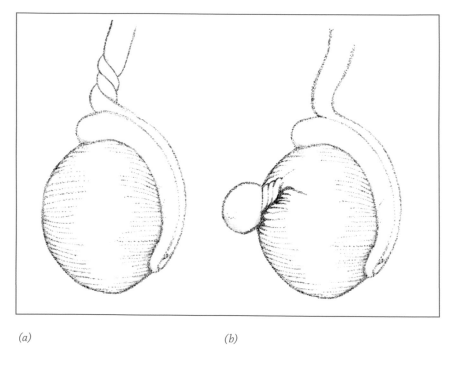

(a)   (b)

Figure 2.1: Torsion of the spermatic cord (a) and torted hydatid of Morgagni (b)

Various clinical signs have been described to help confirm or exclude torsion of the spermatic cord. However, in the authors' experience, such signs are rarely useful. The examination should include an abdominal examination and focussed scrotal examination assessing the testes for: symmetry, lie, size, tenderness, any epididymal abnormality and any skin changes (such as overlying scrotal erythema). Occasionally in young children, a blue discoloration may be visible directly overlying a tender torted hydatid. In the young child presenting with abdominal pain, it is crucial to assess the testes as they may have testicular torsion. Blood tests are seldom useful but a urinalysis is helpful, particularly if the history and examination is suggestive of an infection. As with any emergency patient, a full set of observations is essential.

Urological teaching is that if torsion is suspected, or there is any doubt as to the diagnosis, then urgent exploration is required. This involves a careful consent process. The possibilities of unilateral/bilateral scrotal fixation or orchidectomy need to be explained. As the on-call doctor, you will need to book theatres and discuss the case with the on-call anaesthetist. The patient must also be correctly marked but it is crucial that the operating surgeon reviews the patient him-/herself prior to theatre and takes time to ensure that the patient and parents understand the possibilities of surgical management.

Acute epididymo-orchitis can present with acute scrotal pain and these patients may well undergo urgent testicular exploration if there is a doubt over the diagnosis. The management requires urinalysis, advice to visit a genito-urinary medicine clinic and antibiotics (typically fluoroquinolone +/- doxycycline in younger patients). An US scan is helpful to confirm the diagnosis, exclude a testicular abscess and rule out a testicular tumour.

EMERGENCY DEPARTMENT

2.3 HAEMATURIA

Haematuria can be visible or non-visible (i.e. only detectable on urinalysis). Most hospitals have a designated haematuria clinic where patients can be seen rapidly and investigated for haematuria as an outpatient. In a stable patient with no evidence of urinary retention/voiding difficulties, a referring GP can be directed to this service as such presentations can be managed on an outpatient basis.

The most common indications for admission and inpatient management are clot retention and anaemia in patients with known bladder cancer. Assessment of the emergency patient with haematuria requires a rapid clinical assessment of airway, breathing and circulation to ensure haemodynamic and respiratory stability. Key points from the history include previous episodes, loin, back or bone pain, family history of urological malignancy, anticoagulation and trauma. Intravenous access, with blood samples sent for FBC, U&E and clotting studies, is important. Furthermore, a G&S sample will enable the rapid provision of cross-matched blood if required. A full abdominal examination including DRE is essential and a PSA blood test may also be indicated.

Clot retention requires prompt insertion of a large catheter (ideally a 22Ch 3-way) to enable a thorough bladder washout to be performed. This requires a 50ml bladder tipped syringe and sterile saline/water to attempt to extract any clots. To reduce the risk of bladder rupture, it is important always to aspirate from the catheter prior to infusing fluid. Only once this is achieved should irrigation be commenced using a urology irrigation set to maximise flow.

The bladder is unusual in that if clots persist in the bladder, the haematuria will not settle. If, despite vigorous washouts with irrigation, the bleeding continues, the patient may well require an emergency general anaesthetic cystoscopy and bladder washout in theatre. It can also be useful to involve a haematologist, particularly if anticoagulation needs reversing or platelet consumption is occurring due to the on-going bleeding. Monitor haemoglobin levels and ensure any coagulopathy is corrected. Upper urinary tract imaging is crucial to ensure the bleeding is not coming from the kidneys, with CT urography being the gold standard.

2.4 URINARY TRACT INFECTION (UTI) AND SEPSIS

UTI is the inflammatory response of the urothelium to a micro-organism. This is most commonly bacterial, with gram negative organisms being the likely culprits (E. Coli, Proteus, Klebsiella). Specific questions regarding duration of symptoms, fever, immune compromise (including diabetes mellitus), abnormal urinary tracts and in-dwelling catheters are crucial.

TOP TIP:

When referred a patient, try to classify the UTI into the following categories:

- Uncomplicated and complicated (those occurring in a structurally abnormal urinary tract),

- Upper or lower (history of loin pain suggestive of pyelonephritis versus suprapubic suggestive of cystitis) and

- Isolated, persistent or recurrent (reinfection with the same or different bacteria respectively).

Uncomplicated UTIs can be managed in the community. Complicated UTIs may require emergency admission. It is therefore crucial to take a full history and examination including a urinalysis, sending the sample for microscopy, culture and sensitivity. Vital signs will help to identify a 'septic patient' (the systemic inflammatory response syndrome caused by an infection). These patients may require critical care involvement and upper tract imaging to ensure there is no obstruction. The management of urinary sepsis is consistent with the fundamentals of caring for a septic patient. These include oxygen, IV fluid resuscitation, urinary catheter, blood and urine cultures, a serum lactate level and prompt antibiotics. In a sick patient with confirmed gram-negative sepsis, always consider the possibility of urinary tract obstruction. Urgent imaging of the kidneys will help to identify those patients who may benefit from upper tract decompression.

EMERGENCY DEPARTMENT

2.5 URINARY RETENTION

This is a common urological presentation. Urinary retention can be acute (the painful inability to void in the presence of a painful, percussable bladder) or chronic (the presence of a palpable or percussable bladder in someone who has just voided).

ACUTE URINARY RETENTION (AUR)

This is a urological emergency. After confirming the diagnosis, prompt urethral catheterisation is essential. A 12Ch urethral catheter is adequate. Record the residual (amount initially drained after insertion), perform an abdominal and rectal examination, record vital signs, perform a urine dipstick and send blood for U&E. If residual is less than 1,000ml, the patient is well with no evidence of infection and renal function normal, the patient can be sent home from the emergency department. Remember to consider other diagnoses if the pain persists after catheterisation or the residual is low; don't be caught out by a ruptured abdominal aortic aneurysm being labelled as AUR!

The history should try to differentiate between *precipitated* (constipation, recent surgery, alcohol, drugs) and *spontaneous* AUR. Starting an alpha-blocker (e.g. tamsulosin 400 micrograms once daily) may help to pass a successful trial without catheter (TWOC) which should be booked for the next 1–2 weeks. The majority of AUR fit the above description and will be managed by the ED. Indications for admission include a high residual volume, impaired renal function and, of course, the patient being acutely unwell. Finally, remember that urinary retention can be caused by a variety of non-urological conditions (e.g. pneumonia in the elderly comorbid patient) and in these patients admission under a more appropriate team is advisable.

CHRONIC URINARY RETENTION

This can be normal in a significant proportion of the elderly population and there is no set threshold figure for what is a normal post-void residual in this age group. This means that an asymptomatic individual with normal renal function does not automatically require a catheter if they are found to have a high residual volume. This group of patients can be referred to urology as an outpatient for assessment.

The group of patients you will see is of those with chronic retention but with new onset of renal impairment. These patients may report only mild symptoms, but you must specifically ask about nocturnal bed-wetting and if their trousers/belts are getting tighter. Alternatively, they may be referred to you following an US or CT scan done to investigate deteriorating renal function or an abdominal mass and finding a distended bladder and hydronephrosis. Impaired renal function in this setting is likely to be post-renal and warrants catheterisation. The crucial point in managing this patient sub-group is to watch out for a post-obstructive diuresis. This is usually **physiological** and is caused as the kidneys respond to relief of obstruction by off-loading retained salt and water that have built up during the obstruction. It should settle spontaneously as long as the patient is allowed to eat and drink normally. A small proportion will proceed to develop a **pathological** diuresis, which is caused by the kidney's inability to concentrate urine due to the loss of the cortico-medullary concentration gradient and effects of atrial natriuretic peptide and urea causing an osmotic diuresis. These patients can produce huge quantities of dilute urine per day and it is these patients who require IV fluid (normal saline) replacement at between 50% and 80% of their urine output. These patients can be in hospital for a number of days whilst their kidney function normalises and during this time require daily blood tests, daily weights and hourly urine output. Once the diuresis and renal function have settled, it is important that a trial without catheter (TWOC) is *not* performed: simply removing the catheter will result in the whole situation happening again. The long-term options are: long-term catheterisation, bladder outflow surgery or regular self-catheterisation. The pathophysiology behind the post-obstructive diuresis found in chronic high-pressure retention is the same in any situation where bilateral upper tract obstruction has occurred. This includes retroperitoneal fibrosis, malignant ureteric obstruction and bilateral ureteric calculi. The key is to maintain a high index of suspicion for a pathological diuresis in these patients whilst not over-treating a physiological diuresis.

EMERGENCY DEPARTMENT

2.6 DIFFICULT CATHETERISATION

This is frequently encountered whilst on-call. Male catheterisation can be complicated by a tight foreskin (phimosis – see Figure 2.2a), urethral stricture, enlarged prostate or following prostatic surgery. Difficult female catheters are usually due to overweight patients and difficulty finding the meatus, but occasionally abnormal anatomy or gynaecological malignancy can be the cause.

The first question to ask is "*does the patient definitely require a catheter?*" Frequently, the answer is "*no*". Urine output can be measured by asking the patient to void into a measuring jug; incontinence can be managed using pads/condom sheath collection systems (eg a Conveen®).

> **TOP TIP:**
>
> Always be cautious of the suprapubic mass that has been labelled as an enlarged bladder that persists despite urethral catheterisation as this could represent an undiagnosed pelvic mass.

After confirming that a catheter is required, an attempt with a size 12Ch catheter using sterile conditions is indicated. Always have an assistant, plenty of lubricating jelly and help to expose the meatus in a female. If unsuccessful then try a different size (e.g. 16Ch) as the extra rigidity may help.

If the catheter is not progressing then don't force it because this may cause trauma. At this point you will be asking for some senior help. They may utilise a Tiemann tipped catheter which helps negotiate the prostate, a catheter introducer, a flexible cystoscopy and guidewire, or even a suprapubic catheter. These are specialist skills and untrained doctors should not use an introducer/flexible cystoscopy without guidance. Various catheterisation techniques will be introduced in Chapter 6

> **TOP TIP:**
>
> If unsuccessful when attempting a 'difficult catheter' in a female patient, try keeping the catheter in place whilst attempting with a new one. This will prevent you from inserting it into the incorrect place as before and sometimes a number of catheters can be required until the urethral meatus is identified.

BLOCKED CATHETER

Catheters can become blocked for a variety of reasons. Often this can be resolved by flushing the catheter, so it is wise to check if this has been done in the first instance. After that you can suggest the host team change the catheter to a new one and see if that improves things. Make sure they are confident it is in the correct place as sometimes you may find the catheter tip can sit in the prostatic urethra (in males) or vagina (in females) rather than in the bladder. If the catheter has become blocked after haematuria was noticed, it might be sensible to consider changing it to a 3-way catheter (see Figure 1.4) and performing a thorough bladder washout.

A DISLODGED SUPRAPUBIC CATHETER (SPC)

If an SPC has fallen out, the most important question is how long has it been out for? Established SPC tracks that have been there for years can stay open for several hours provided the patient hasn't mobilised. The tracks close over when the patient moves/coughs/sneezes and the abdominal layers slide over and obstruct the tract. If only a short time has passed, you might be able to reinsert it. If the referring team has tried but been unsuccessful, you should attempt it yourself, but you are likely to have the same result. Speak to your senior as they may be able to pass a guidewire and then dilate the tract to enable a catheter to be re-inserted.

The next thing is to place a urethral catheter for the patient. This will protect their bladder in the short term and arrangements can be made by you for an elective SPC insertion either under cystoscopic or US guidance. In the less common circumstance that a urethral catheter cannot be inserted, ask your senior to inspect the urethra with a flexible cystoscope (as you can sometimes place a catheter this way with a guidewire). Failing that, the patient will need an US-guided SPC insertion: you will need to coordinate a radiologist to provide US support and your senior to place the SPC for you. Alternatively, admit the patient until they develop a palpable bladder, at which point reinserting an SPC becomes less risky.

2.7 PARAPHIMOSIS

This condition arises where a foreskin has been retracted and cannot be replaced over the glans. A constricting band causes venous and lymphatic oedema resulting in an increasingly swollen prepuce (Figure 2.2b). If left for long enough, the band or even the glans can become ischaemic and necrotic, with subsequent infection being a significant problem. The management of acute paraphimosis requires a careful explanation to an often very anxious patient as to the underlying problem. Resolution requires squeezing the oedema out of the glans and then replacing the constricting band back over the glans. Frequently, this is not done properly and patients have been reassured the paraphimosis has been fixed where in fact the constricting band is still in place below the coronal sulcus. You may require a penile block using local anaesthetic (combination of 1% lidocaine and 0.5% Marcaine without adrenaline, remembering the terminal artery blood supply to the penis and risk of penile necrosis if adrenaline is used (see section 6.5)). This provides excellent anaesthesia which permits additional force or rarely a dorsal slit to be employed. This involves an incision with a blade into the constricting phimotic band under sterile conditions with surgical prep and drape. Following reduction, it is sensible to arrange an outpatient review as some (but not all) of these patients may require a circumcision.

In patients with a long-term catheter, a 'chronic paraphimosis' can develop where the foreskin remains retracted without constriction and the prepuce will not stay in a retracted position. These can be left alone.

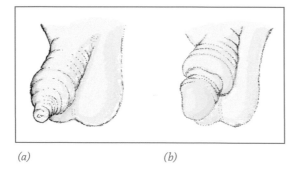

(a)   (b)

Figure 2.2: Diagram illustrating (a) phimosis and (b) para-phimosis. A **phimosis** is a tight constricted opening to the foreskin (arrow) which does not retract. This is common in children (physiological) and usually resolves with age. In older patients, it may be related to BXO (balanitis xerotica obliterans) which can require a circumcision. A **paraphimosis** is where the foreskin has been retracted and cannot be replaced. An oedematous, swollen "ring" develops which makes the situation worse. There is usually a constricted band of foreskin proximally which must be fully replaced over the glans.

2.8 UROLOGICAL TRAUMA

The American Association for the Surgery of Trauma has a detailed classification of many aspects of urological trauma, on which we have broadly based our management of urological trauma below.

RENAL

The majority of renal trauma presenting to ED is blunt, although penetrating trauma is increasing. Iatrogenic trauma is usually identified intra- or post-operatively. Any trauma patient should be managed according to advanced trauma life support (ATLS) principles as part of a trauma team with an "ABCDE" approach. Basics including vital signs, oxygen, IV access and baseline bloods, including G&S, are essential. You should suspect renal injury with any mechanism involving sudden deceleration or significant force. The kidney is mobile on its vascular pedicle and a sudden stop can risk injury. The majority of renal injuries, such as those shown in Figure 2.3, are identified following a trauma series CT scan. This will provide good detail of the renal parenchyma but will not include a delayed urographic phase. This is crucial in detecting any disruption to the collecting system and subsequent urinary extravasation.

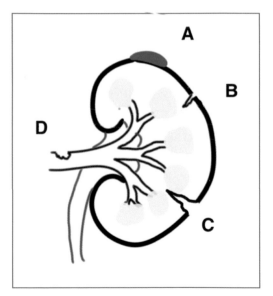

Figure 2.3: The variation of renal trauma. Minor injuries involve contusions or subscapular haematomas (A). Renal parenchymal injuries can vary in size, some remaining superficial (B) while some extend further towards the urinary collecting system (C) and can cause urinary extravasation. Multiple injuries to the renal tissue can lead to shattering of the kidney, with the loss of typical renal anatomy, while vascular injury to the renal vessels (D) is also a risk, along with avulsion of the hilum.

EMERGENCY DEPARTMENT

The majority of renal trauma will be managed non-operatively and if intervention is required this is usually in the form of angio-embolisation. Emergency nephrectomy is thankfully a rare procedure but can be necessary. When referred a renal injury, rapidly review the patient and ensure that the basics from an ATLS approach have been done (e.g. cervical spine clearance). Early involvement of your on-call senior is important as renal trauma can be life-threatening. Penetrating renal trauma is rare. Rarely, in an unstable patient a renal injury may not be identified until reaching the operating theatre. Again, your seniors are going to be involved at this point but it is important to remember that, in this setting, an on-table IVU is required to ensure the contra-lateral kidney is functioning well. An IV contrast dose of 1mg/kg is used. Indications for a CT scan to assess a possible renal injury include blunt trauma with visible haematuria or non-visible haematuria and haemodynamic instability, patients with a history of rapid deceleration and penetrating trauma.

BLADDER

Bladder trauma should be suspected with blunt trauma, lower abdominal pain and haematuria. Classical presentation is of an alcoholic who falls onto a full bladder causing a bladder rupture or a patient in a road traffic accident where the mechanism compresses a full bladder again the dashboard/steering wheel. Prompt imaging is essential. For a conventional cystogram, it is important to fill the bladder to 150–300ml with contrast and to take post-emptying films (including at oblique angles). If a CT cystogram is available, it may be performed instead of a conventional cystogram.

URETHRAL

Suspect a urethral injury with a relevant mechanism (e.g. fall astride injury or kick to perineum) associated with difficulty voiding and haematuria. The posterior urethra is vulnerable in major trauma cases with pelvic fractures. If a urethral injury is suspected then involve your on-call senior. A gentle attempt at urethral catheterisation is appropriate, but if any resistance is met then a urethrogram proceeding to either cystoscopic-guided urethral catheterisation or an SPC for urinary diversion may be required.

GENITAL

Trauma to the external genitalia can affect the penis or scrotum. Penile fracture refers to a tear in the tunica albuginea which surrounds the erectile tissue of the corpora cavernosa. Patients describe an audible "pop" or a "click" during intercourse followed by rapid detumescence. The penis will swell and be bruised, giving the "aubergine sign". It is crucial to ask if the patient has voided and, if so, whether there was any haematuria, as 10–20% of penile fractures may have an associated urethral injury. Treatment is surgical but this can usually be performed the following morning. Treatment aims are to reduce deformity in the long term but patients need to be made aware of the risk of long-term erectile dysfunction.

PENILE AMPUTATION

Fortunately, this is very rare but frequently associated with psychiatric pathology and patients can be difficult to manage. Don't underestimate the degree of blood loss that may have occurred. Treatment requires IV access, G&S, resuscitation and control of haemorrhage. Following this, microvascular anastomosis should be considered in a specialist centre.

SCROTAL TRAUMA

This can be blunt or penetrating. Blunt trauma may be a kick to the testis or direct impact with a ball during sports. The important differentiating point is whether there is a testicular rupture. A prompt scrotal US can help to demonstrate this, and even if a tear in the tunica is not visualised, the finding of a heterogenous appearance to the testes warrants exploration to debride any devascularised tubules and repair the tunica albuginea. Patients and their relatives need to be aware of the risk of an orchidectomy and contra-lateral testis fixation if the testis is not salvageable. If there is no rupture of the tunica albuginea then conservative management with analgesia, scrotal support and antibiotics is appropriate.

EMERGENCY DEPARTMENT

2.9 PRIAPISM

This is a prolonged erection. It can be classified into ischaemic (low-flow) or non-ischaemic (high-flow). The most common type is ischaemic, which is painful and results in congestion of the erectile tissue with blood. Key points from the history are: previous episodes, sickle cell disease, haematological problems/malignancy, drug use (both illicit and prescribed), erectile dysfunction treatments, pelvic malignancy, trauma and duration of symptoms. Examination is usually obvious but in non-ischaemic priapism the penis may not be fully erect.

ISCHAEMIC PRIAPISM

Send a baseline FBC and clotting screen and, if indicated, a sickle cell screen. Initial management includes analgesia and asking the patient to mobilise/walk up and down stairs. The practicalities of this are often a bit more challenging to manage and frequently the patient has tried this prior to coming to ED. The next step is to administer a penile block and then to aspirate blood from the corpora with a green butterfly needle placed laterally into the penile shaft. This can also be performed on the opposite side with an aim to aspirate the congested blood from the erectile tissue. This may well be successful and if so, it is sensible to observe the patient afterwards to ensure it does not return. If this fails then it is advisable to involve your on-call senior.

Patients will need to be in a monitored bed, usually in ED resus and phenylephrine is used to bring on detumescence. Take a 10mg/ml vial of phenylephrine from the on-call anaesthetist and dilute it in 19ml of normal saline. This gives a 0.5mg/ml solution. Proceed to give 0.5ml aliquots (250 micrograms of phenylephrine) every 5 mins INTRA-CAVERNOSALLY, ensuring that the patient's pulse and blood pressure remain stable. If this fails then your on-call senior is likely to be liaising with a tertiary andrology unit to get advice regarding types of shunts, something beyond the scope of this book. The concern with prolonged priapism is the long-term risk of permanent erectile dysfunction. The corpora becomes replaced with fibrotic tissue after 12–24 hours and there is increasing use of an implantable penile prosthesis in patients with priapism which has persisted for 24–48 hours to aid subsequent management.

NON-ISCHAEMIC PRIAPISM

This is rare and is associated with pelvic trauma leading to an arterio-venous fistula causing continued arterial blood to enter the corpora. This is not an emergency and can be managed with selective angio-embolisation.

EMERGENCY
DEPARTMENT

2.10 UROLOGICAL ISSUES IN PREGNANCY

Managing urological problems in pregnancy is complicated by:

1. Physiological changes
2. Limited availability of investigations and medications
3. Stent/nephrostomy encrustation due to hypercalciuria of pregnancy
4. Logistical challenges.

The two most common situations encountered during pregnancy are loin pain with hydronephrosis and urinary tract infections including pyelonephritis. It is preferable for pregnant women to be managed jointly with the obstetric team and it is the authors' preference that they are sited on a women's health ward with urological involvement, for the reasons listed above.

HYDRONEPHROSIS OF PREGNANCY

Pregnancy can result in physiological hydronephrosis. This is more common on the right than the left and tends to occur onwards from 20 weeks. It is multifactorial but causes include ureteric compression by the uterus and progesterone-induced ureteric dilation. In a pregnant lady with loin pain the initial investigation is an US. However, the finding of hydronephrosis could be either physiological or pathological (a ureteric calculus). A urine dipstick to look for non-visible haematuria is helpful. If the pain settles then conservative management with early outpatient review is indicated. If it doesn't then a decision regarding further imaging (MR urography is thought to be safe in the second and third trimesters, although some units might employ ultra-low-dose CT KUB) or intervention (stent or nephrostomy) is required. This will involve senior members of the obstetric and urology team. The concern with any stent or nephrostomy is that rapid encrustation requires them to be changed regularly.

ASYMPTOMATIC BACTERIURIA

This is present in up to 10% of pregnant women and associated with a 20–40% risk of developing pyelonephritis. Pyelonephritis can result in a very unwell patient with risk to the baby. It is for this reason that asymptomatic bacteriuria should be treated in pregnant women.

TOP TIP:

Trimethoprim and nitrofurantoin are contra-indicated in pregnancy.

Amoxicillin and cephalexin are the most commonly used oral antibiotics. Ensure that the urine becomes sterile following treatment. In the emergency situation with a septic patient with a presumed pyelonephritis, an US KUB scan is useful to identify hydronephrosis and plan an emergency percutaneous nephrostomy.

EMERGENCY
DEPARTMENT

2.11 ASSESSING A POST-OPERATIVE PATIENT FOR URETERIC INJURY

Iatrogenic urological trauma can be encountered following treatment from a variety of specialities. The important principle is always to consider the possibility of damage to a ureter when a patient who has undergone any pelvic procedure presents with loin pain, fever, increased drain output or leakage of clear fluid through the vagina or perineum. Send the fluid off for a fluid creatinine. If it is urine, the result will be very high. If it is the same as the serum creatinine then it is not urine.

> **TOP TIP:**
>
> Operations during which ureteric/bladder injury may occur more frequently include:
>
> • Hysterectomy
>
> • Continence procedures
>
> • Colorectal procedures
>
> • Ureteroscopy.

Managing these patients is complicated and has significant medico-legal implications. Involve your on-call senior early. Sensible discussion with the operating surgeons, explanation to the patient and careful documentation are vital. A CT urogram is usually helpful but a cystoscopy with bilateral retrogrades is the optimal diagnostic test. Although the subsequent management is complex and beyond the scope of this book, briefly, early recognition in a well patient should allow an acute repair. However, a delayed recognition (usually >14 days) or where patients are unwell, it is often better to manage with temporary drainage (e.g. nephrostomy) with a delayed definitive repair after 2-3 months.

EMERGENCY DEPARTMENT

2.12 PAEDIATRICS

The main paediatric presentations to the ED will relate to the acute scrotum, foreskin problems (phimosis and paraphimosis), urinary retention and trauma. Testicular torsion, acute epididymo-orchitis and testicular rupture have already been described.

SCROTAL SWELLING

Always consider an acute presentation of an inguino-scrotal hernia and/or patent processus vaginalis (PPV) in your differential. The latter is usually well described by the child's parent, who might report a painless intermittent testicular swelling. The diagnosis is confirmed by the finding of a painless hydrocele which trans-illuminates. This can be managed with an elective procedure to ligate the PPV.

ACUTE URINARY RETENTION IN CHILDREN

Rarely, you may be asked to see a young boy with balanoposthitis who has difficulty voiding due to pain/inflammation of his foreskin. Although difficult, it is important to reassure the boy's parents that things will invariably settle with antibiotics/analgesics, and encouragement to void whilst in a warm bath will usually work. Involve the paediatric nursing staff and make sure the child voids with a check post-void scan before they are discharged. It is very rare to have to catheterise a boy with balanoposthitis. If there is no abnormality with the foreskin, then consider seeking specialist paediatric urological advice to further investigate rare but sinister causes (e.g. prostate rhabdomyosarcoma).

RENAL TRAUMA

The kidneys are more vulnerable to trauma in children than in adults due to increased mobility and reduced perinephric fat. Take seriously any child who presents with a significant mechanism of injury or with abdominal/loin pain following an injury and haematuria. Prompt assessment adhering to ATLS principles and imaging (see 'Urological trauma' section) is essential.

EMERGENCY DEPARTMENT

CHAPTER 3: THE WARD

3.1 THE WARD ROUND

The key to a harmonious start to the day is an efficient ward round. The majority of patients will be located on the main urology ward (if your hospital is lucky enough to have one!). However, urology consults are commonly sought on medical patients for a host of reasons such as urinary retention, incidental renal tumours, renal failure and haematuria post anticoagulation/thrombolysis. As such, at any given time some of your patients will be found as outliers on medical and non-urological surgery wards. Being organised and up to date will save a lot of time and stress. A meticulous, thorough and up-to-date list of patients with pertinent clinical information (such as presenting complaint, past medical history, results of investigations and treatment provided) will go a long way to ensuring all patients are reviewed in a timely manner.

3.2 PRESCRIBING INTRAVENOUS FLUIDS

You will be called to give IV fluids in a variety of scenarios, such as the peri-operative period, post-obstructive diuresis or in those acutely unwell patients requiring fluid resuscitation (e.g. sepsis or haemorrhage). It should not be forgotten that all IV fluid regimes need careful consideration and planning.

Water requirements

As a guide, an unstressed healthy adult requires 30–40ml/kg/day.

For an average male of 70kg, that equates to approximately 2.1–2.8L/day.

Electrolyte requirements

When prescribing fluids, your primary electrolyte considerations are sodium and potassium:

   Na^+ 2mmol/kg/day

   K^+ 1mmol/kg/day

Your decision to start fluids and what fluids to give should be based on a combination of clinical and biochemical evidence. A thorough assessment of a patient's fluid balance and overall hydration, taking note of mucous membranes, JVP, urine output (0.5ml/kg/hr), central and peripheral oedema, and on-going fluid losses is fundamental to fluid resuscitation. Always check a patient's recent biochemistry results before initiating fluid therapy.

INTRAVENOUS FLUID PRODUCTS

Fluids are described as either being crystalloid or colloid. Crystalloid fluids contain electrolytes, whereas colloid fluids contain high molecular weight molecules to mimic the colloid osmotic effect of large plasma proteins (albumin) raising intravascular volume. As such, colloids have been favoured in resuscitation of shocked patients (e.g. acute hypovolaemia), although recent evidence shows no difference between crystalloid and colloid resuscitation in the acute/short-term setting. For correcting electrolyte imbalance and fluid maintenance, crystalloids are the fluid of choice. In the context of overt haemorrhage, the optimal product of choice should be packed red cells.

> **TOP TIP:**
>
> **So how much fluid should I prescribe?**
>
> Commonly, patients will require 1–2L of IV fluid peri-operatively to keep them hydrated. For prolonged periods, patients require carefully prescribed fluid maintenance regimes.

NORMAL FLUID MAINTENANCE

The regimes below are based on an average 70kg adult. Your regime can be adapted accordingly to account for variable patient factors.

Regimen A

- 1L normal saline 0.9%   over 8 hours   plus 20mmol K^+
- 1L 5% dextrose   over 8 hours   plus 20mmol K^+
- 1L 5% dextrose   over 8 hours   plus 20mmol K^+

Total = 3,000ml with 154mmol Na^+ and 60mmol K^+

Regimen B

- 1L Hartmann's solution   over 8 hours
- 1L Hartmann's solution   over 8 hours
- 1L Hartmann's solution   over 8 hours

Total = 3,000ml with 393mmol Na^+ and 15mmol K^+

Hartmann's solution, otherwise known as Ringer's lactate, is the most physiological solution and most isotonic with blood. It is therefore recommended for use as the first-line fluid choice if available. It may not be suitable for prolonged use to meet daily requirements of sodium and potassium intake as 15mmol K+ in a 24hr period isn't sufficient on a prolonged basis.

THE WARD

3.3 POST-OBSTRUCTIVE DIURESIS

Post-obstructive diuresis is a polyuric response initiated by the kidneys after the relief of a substantial bladder outlet obstruction. In severe cases this condition can become pathological, resulting in dehydration, electrolyte imbalances and death if not adequately treated.

Patients who have a residual volume of more than 1L with renal impairment are at risk. These patients should have the following:

- Urinary catheter insertion, left on free drainage (do not clamp the catheter)
- Daily weights
- Daily urea and electrolytes check
- Lying and standing blood pressure
- Hourly urine output measures
- Encourage oral fluid rehydration
- If the urine output is > 200ml/hr for two consecutive hours, institute IV fluid replacement with normal saline. The rate of administration should be prescribed such that 50% of the preceding hour's output is replaced in the next hour and so on.

For example, if from 1pm to 2pm urine output equals 400ml, then 200ml of IV fluid will need to be administered from 3pm to 4pm.

Table 3.1: Management of post-obstructive diuresis

THE WARD

3.4 PATIENTS WITH ABNORMAL BLOOD GLUCOSE

HYPOGLYCAEMIA

Many of the urology patients seen during on-calls will be susceptible to this, including:

- Diabetics – in particular insulin-dependent diabetics
- Elderly patients
- Septic patients
- Patients having undergone periods of starvation either pre- or post-operatively.

Hypoglycaemia is a blood glucose of less than 4mmol/L. If the patient is asymptomatic, repeat the test. Ideally, confirm with a lab sample. **Do NOT wait for the result – treat at once.**

Clinical presentation of hypoglycaemia:

4mmol/L　　Patient is conscious and able to swallow. Trembling, sweating, hungry, tingling, headache, anxiety, palpitations, nausea, forgetfulness.

2–3mmol/L　Patient is conscious and able to swallow but in need of assistance. Difficulty in concentrating, speaking, confusion, weakness, drowsiness, unsteady, headache.

<1.5mmol/L　Patient is unconscious and unable to swallow. Fitting.

MANAGEMENT

If the patient is alert and able to swallow:
- Oral glucose, e.g. Glucotabs™, Lucozade™ or fruit juice
- Give long-acting carbohydrate such as toast
- Re-assess patient.

If the patient is unwell/unresponsive or unable to swallow:
- 100ml of 10% glucose IV
- If no IV access, give 1mg IM glucagon
- Re-assess patient, continue to monitor blood glucose levels, repeat if necessary
- Consider transfer to ITU.

THE WARD

> **TOP TIP:**
>
> *Never omit insulin following an episode. Involve the endocrine or medical team* ***early****.*

HYPERGLYCAEMIA

The stress response to sepsis and surgery creates a hyperglycaemic state related to the hypermetabolic stress response to cortisol which increases glucose production and causes insulin resistance. The most important diagnosis in patients with elevated blood glucose is to exclude diabetic ketoacidosis (DKA) or hyperosmolar hyperglycaemic state (HHS). In patients with persistently high glucose, always consult your senior or the medical/endocrine team.

WHAT TO DO WITH DIABETIC PATIENTS BEFORE SURGERY

Aim to put any diabetic patient first on the operating list.

Pre-operative assessment

- Patients with type 2 diabetes managed with diet alone need no intervention prior to surgery.
- For procedures involving intravenous radio-contrast, discontinue metformin 48 hours prior to the procedure.

Before surgery

- To ensure that blood glucose is controlled within normal limits before surgery (target range: 5–10mmol/L), a random blood glucose should be obtained soon after the patient is admitted. If it is not within the target range, advice should be sought from the diabetic team, the anaesthetic team or both.
- Patients should receive their usual doses of oral hypoglycaemic and/or insulin (except for long-acting) on the day prior to surgery, including evening doses. For long-acting insulin, normal evening doses should be modified (often halved, but check with your local protocol) and then given with the evening meal. From 6am on the morning of surgery, maintain glycaemic control by starting a glucose/potassium/insulin (GKI) regimen or "sliding scale".

N.B. Always consult your local hospital guidelines.

Post-operative management

Blood glucose measurements should be taken hourly until the reading is stable and within normal range. The first meal following surgery should be eaten while the infusion continues. If tolerated, patients on subcutaneous insulin or oral hypoglycaemics can return to their usual regimen. It is common practice to stop IV insulin infusions soon after the first dose of subcutaneous insulin. For patients taking metformin who receive contrast media, metformin is usually restarted 48 hours after the procedure.

THE WARD

3.5 ANTICOAGULATION

It is increasingly common to find patients on anticoagulants and/or antiplatelet agents. They are usually on these to manage their atrial fibrillation, to prevent thromboses or because they have mechanical heart valves. The majority of urology patients will require their anticoagulation to be withheld and heparin prescribed until two hours pre-operatively. However, in some circumstances such as emergency ureteric stenting to relieve obstruction secondary to a ureteric stone, no anticoagulation reversal is required.

Below is a list of commonly used anticoagulants and peri-operative modifications to their use (Table 3.2). You should have a low threshold to seek cardiology advice in the context of recently inserted coronary stents as these patients are often on dual antiplatelet therapy and omission may be hazardous. Restarting anticoagulation after surgery should be directed by the operating surgeon. This requires balancing the risks of bleeding with the benefits of VTE reduction. Haematology may need to be consulted. Remember that patients at risk of thromboembolism will need further post-operative heparin until the INR is within therapeutic range.

Anticoagulant/ antiplatelet	Mechanism of action	Number of days to stop prior to surgery	Reversal	Notes
Warfarin	Vitamin K antagonist	5	Vitamin K or prothrombin complex concentrate	Check INR before surgery; if <1.3, it is often considered safe to proceed.
Clopidogrel	Platelet inhibitor	7	Platelets	
Ticagrelor	Inhibits platelet aggregation	7	Platelets	
Rivaroxaban	Factor Xa inhibitor	2	No reversal available	
Dipyridamole	Inhibits platelet function	7	Platelets	
Aspirin	Inhibits platelet function	5	Platelets	

Table 3.2: Anticoagulant/antiplatelet agents

THE WARD

3.6 NEPHROSTOMIES AND ABDOMINAL DRAINS

A nephrostomy is a drain inserted into the collecting system of the kidney either to relieve obstruction or temporarily to divert urine away from the lower urinary tract. Indications for nephrostomy insertion include:

- Relief of distal obstruction, e.g. ureteric stone, malignant extra mural compression
- Following percutaneous nephrolithotomy (PCNL).

A nephrostomy inserted in a collecting system that also has a ureteric stent in situ should be removed by a radiologist under fluoroscopic guidance to avoid stent migration. If there is no stent, a nephrostomy can be safely removed on the ward after unlocking the mechanism keeping the 'J-curl' of the nephrostomy in place.

Abdominal drains are commonly left in situ following pelvic oncological surgery such as prostatectomy and cystectomy. Instructions on removal are typically cited in the operation note instructions. If in doubt, contact the operating surgeon. As a general rule abdominal drains can be removed once the output is less than 100ml in 24hrs, although each surgeon will have a preference.

N.B. If the output from a drain looks suspiciously like urine, send the contents to the lab for creatinine level assessment. If it is urine, the result will be very high. If it is the same as the serum creatinine then it is not urine. Patients can become unwell, and urgent senior urological opinion is required.

THE WARD

3.7 CATHETERS AND IRRIGATION

Catheters and bladder irrigation are the mainstay of ward urological management. Catheters can be 2-way or 3-way in nature (see 'Instruments in urology' section). The volume of water in the catheter balloon commonly ranges between 10ml and 50ml. This has important implications on removal. Always check the catheter insertion documentation for how much water is in the balloon as well as timing of the trial without catheter (TWOC). An underinflated balloon during catheter removal can lead to significant urethral trauma.

Irrigation sets and 3-way catheters are used to washout haematuria. Irrigation only stops a new blood clot from forming, and will not remove large quantities of old blood clots. Before establishing bladder irrigation, it is crucial to perform a thorough manual bladder washout (see 'Instruments in urology' section). This will remove old clots, allowing the irrigation to prevent new clots from forming.

THE WARD

3.8 EVALUATING THE ACUTELY "UNWELL" PATIENT

The assessment and management of the acutely unwell urology patient is best achieved using an "ABCDE" approach. A rapid assessment coupled with instituting initial management will save valuable time. Most hospitals host an induction course for assessing acutely unwell patients. It is imperative that you attend such a course, given the frequency of such referrals and the positive impact that can be made during the initial stages.

Often, a severely unwell patient is described as "shocked". Physiologically, the term "shock" relates to "an abnormality of the circulatory system that results in inadequate organ perfusion and tissue oxygenation."

Signs of shock include:
- Tachycardia (heart rate > 100 beats/minute)
- Hypotension (systolic blood pressure < 100mmHg)
- Tachypnoea (respiratory rate > 20 breaths/minute)
- Decreased urine output
- Altered mental status.

In urology, the common acute scenarios are septic shock (e.g. obstructed kidney) and hypovolaemic shock (e.g. secondary to haemorrhage following transurethral resection of the prostate (TURP)).

AIRWAY

Is the airway patent? Can the patient speak in full sentences? Are there upper airway noises?

Give oxygen 15L/min through a non-rebreathable mask with the reservoir bag ready-inflated.

If you feel the patient is unable to maintain his or her airway, call a crash team immediately. In the meantime, attempt the following to improve and maintain the airway:

1) Airway manoeuvre: chin lift or jaw thrust
2) Airway adjunct: Guedel oropharyngeal airway or a nasopharyngeal airway
3) Semi-definitive airway: laryngeal mask airway
4) Definitive airway: intubation performed by an anaesthetist.

THE WARD

BREATHING

- Inspection and palpate chest movements, percuss for dullness
- Auscultate for breath sounds in all zones: superior, middle and inferior zones bilaterally
- Assess the respiratory rate and oxygen saturation
- Further investigations will be guided by the history and your findings (e.g. chest radiograph, arterial blood gas, computed tomography pulmonary angiogram (CTPA)).

N.B. Pulmonary embolus (e.g. from prothrombotic states such as dehydration, malignancy and immobility), chest infection and fluid overload are common post-operative findings in urology patients. A thorough awareness of the diagnosis and management should be appreciated.

CIRCULATION

- Assess heart rate, blood pressure and urine output (normal > 0.5ml/kg/hr)
- Obtain the patient's temperature; consider early IV or oral antibiotics
- Gain IV access and take blood for: culture (if pyrexial), full blood count, urea and electrolytes, c-reactive protein, coagulation studies, group and save
- Give IV fluid challenges if signs of shock.

DISABILITY

- Assessment of the patient's neurological disability using the Glasgow Coma Score. Look for causes such as hypoglycaemia, sedatives, analgesics and electrolyte disturbances.
- Any patient with acute cognitive impairment should be closely monitored with neuro-observations for any further deterioration.
- If the cause of decreased consciousness is not immediately obvious and reversible (e.g. opioids or hypoglycaemia), contact the on-call senior team for advice.

EXPOSURE

- Assess the patient for any external injuries such as open fractures and wounds.

THE WARD

3.9 COMMON POST-OPERATIVE PROBLEMS

Below is a list of commonly performed procedures within urology departments and associated ward-based complications that the on-call junior team will be asked to manage. This is a guide and each urology senior will have a different approach to managing these complications. Liaise with the on-call urology senior early in the management, having conducted a thorough review of the problem: history, examination and commencing basic investigatory/therapeutic measures.

TRANSURETHRAL RESECTION OF THE PROSTATE (TURP)

Following a TURP, you may be called to manage either catheter problems (e.g. blockage, bypassing, heavy haematuria) or post-operative confusion/delirium.

- Catheter problems – the first step is to stop the bladder irrigation and flush the catheter by performing a thorough bladder washout. It may well be that there are residual prostate chips which are blocking the catheter or the bleeding is heavy such that clots are forming. Send an urgent venous haemoglobin to quantify the level of blood loss. Having performed a thorough washout, place the catheter on traction so that the catheter balloon can tamponade bleeding from the prostatic fossa. At this point the patient will require a senior review, and a decision as to whether the patient needs to be taken back to theatre for diathermy will need to be made.

- Confusion – as with any unwell patient, an "ABCDE" approach should be taken. The likely causes are sepsis or TUR syndrome. Sepsis is an early complication, whilst TUR syndrome occurs in the immediate post-operative period. A full set of bloods should be sent, with emphasis on the serum sodium and infective markers. If the sodium is low, TUR syndrome should be suspected and senior ITU input will be required as the condition is potentially fatal. Early recognition and communication with senior colleagues are thus imperative. Management involves diuretics, mannitol and high dependency unit (HDU) observation. If sepsis is the cause then early intravenous antibiotics should be initiated, consulting local microbiology guidelines.

THE WARD

SCROTAL AND PENILE SURGERY

Commonly performed procedures on the scrotum include hydrocele repair, epididymal cyst excision, vasectomy, orchidopexy, incision and drainage of scrotal abscess, and emergency scrotal exploration for suspected testicular torsion. The commonest complications include pain, infection and haematoma formation. Approximately 10% of scrotal procedures are complicated by a haematoma that can often be managed conservatively with analgesia and a scrotal support. If the haematoma is large and particularly tender then open surgical evacuation may be warranted. This is a decision that will be made by the senior urologist on-call; however, it would be expected that analgesia, antibiotics and imaging such as an ultrasound would have been arranged by the on-call junior.

Following a circumcision, it is not uncommon for the recovery nurse to report bleeding around the dressing. It is important to avoid delay in making a clinical assessment. In the majority of cases, applying a local anaesthetic penile block followed by interrupted sutures will resolve the bleeding. However, in a small number of cases, if the bleeding is coming from a deep lying vessel, then re-exploration in theatre will be required. Senior support will be required to make this decision.

PELVIC AND ABDOMINAL SURGERY

Pelvic and abdominal surgery within urology includes oncology operations (nephrectomy, prostatectomy, retro-peritoneal lymph node dissection and cystectomy with either ileal conduit or neo-bladder formation) and some reconstructive procedures. In the early post-operative period, these patients are managed no differently to other surgical patients (i.e. early mobilisation, thromboprophylaxis, antibiotics and close adherence to specific instructions noted by the operating surgeon). Decisions on when to remove drains and catheters should be made by the operating surgeon. In the majority of urology settings, nephrectomy is performed laparoscopically. Patients require 1–2 days of inpatient care. Key considerations are post-operative haemoglobin and optimal analgesia to aid early mobilisation. The same considerations are to be noted for prostatectomy patients, who may have had open, laparoscopic or robot-assisted procedures. In addition, it is vitally important **NOT to remove the urinary catheter** as it aids in the healing of the vesicourethral anastomosis. If there is haematuria with clots, perform a gentle washout. If the catheter blocks and requires replacement with a 3-way catheter, a senior member of the urology team should perform this. Cystectomy patients tend to have a more prolonged hospital admission.

THE WARD

The physiological effects of removing the bladder are greater. Nutrition is important and should be guided by the dieticians and the requests of the operating surgeon as ileus is as an all-too-common finding post-operatively. As such, electrolyte imbalances are often seen and managed accordingly.

TOP TIP:

Do not remove the urinary catheter in post-prostatectomy patients without consulting your on-call senior.

THE WARD

CHAPTER 4: THE CLINIC

Urology has a heavy outpatient clinic workload. Whilst not strictly speaking the remit of the on-call urology junior doctor, it is important that you have an understanding of how to manage the common problems that you will see. This chapter is designed to help you in a general urology clinic and also in an "emergency"-style acute clinic which some departments often run.

4.1 FOLLOW-UP OF ACUTE URETERIC COLIC

Most confirmed cases of ureteric colic will have a follow up appointment arranged for 2-4 weeks. This gives enough time for the stone to pass but ensures that a clinical review with a urologist is close by.

Key points from the consultation are:

- Is the patient still in pain?
- Is there any evidence of infection or deterioration in renal function?
- Have they passed the stone? (If they have, send it for analysis.)
- Is this their first episode of colic or are they a recurrent stone former?

Generally speaking, a patient with his/her first episode of colic is discharged if the answers to all the above questions are stable. The best ways to prove that the stone has been passed is either for the patient to confirm that they have passed it or to repeat imaging. This can be either a plain X-ray KUB (if it was visible on the scout film of the CT/X-ray KUB on admission) or a follow-up CT KUB if distal. For some patients, especially younger ones, a follow-up US KUB may suffice. If the stone is still present then intervention may be required, although you will be liaising with you senior about this. It is helpful to send a serum calcium and uric acid level as a baseline screening tool for underlying metabolic problems. For recurrent stone formers, it is safest for them to be under regular follow-up to try to intervene before any stones become symptomatic.

Interventions for renal/ureteric stone disease can be divided into: lithotripsy; ureteroscopy and laser fragmentation; or percutaneous nephrolithotomy. The choice between each approach is beyond the scope of this book but most ureteric stones you will see in an "acute" clinic will either be managed by waiting for them to pass spontaneously, lithotripsy or ureteroscopy. As a result, make sure you ask about any contra-indications to those techniques (e.g. history of anticoagulants, pregnancy and history of abdominal aortic aneurysm).

THE CLINIC

4.2 SCROTAL SWELLINGS

This is a very common reason for a referral into urology. The vast majority of scrotal swellings do not represent a serious underlying pathology but always remember the possibility of a testicular tumour. The history is usually straightforward but key points to ask about are:

- Duration
- Side
- History of previous scrotal swelling, surgery or un-descended testes (this is a risk factor for testicular cancer)
- Impact on quality of life
- Fertility (any scrotal surgery carries a small risk of damage to the vas/ gonadal vessels).

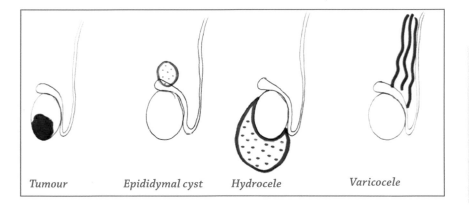

Tumour   Epididymal cyst   Hydrocele   Varicocele

Figure 4.1: Schematic representation of the common scrotal swellings (testicular tumour, epididymal cyst, hydrocele and varicocele)

A testicular tumour will usually present as a firm mass within the testes. Organise an US testes in clinic and if this confirms your clinical suspicion then an urgent radical orchidectomy is required along with tumour markers (hCG, AFP, LDH) and a staging CT chest/abdomen/pelvis. Counselling about a testicular prosthesis, semen banking and an introduction to a urology nurse specialist who can act as their key worker are important. Be aware of the rare situation where a patient with testicular cancer presents with extensive metastatic disease. This requires urgent oncology input and likely hospital admission.

THE CLINIC

Other common scrotal swellings you may see include hydrocele, epididymal cyst and varicocele. A hydrocele is an abnormal amount of fluid between the visceral and parietal layers of the tunica into which the testicle is enveloped. Classically, the testis itself is difficult to palpate and the fluid collection will trans-illuminate. They can be primary (no cause apparent) or secondary (following infection, trauma, tumour, etc). The main indication for intervention is increasing size with associated discomfort and impact on quality of life. They can be repaired surgically as a day case procedure and, in very unfit patients, there is the option of needle aspiration, although the recurrence rate is high.

Epididymal cysts are common and can be single or multiple. The diagnosis is usually apparent on examination, although very large cysts can mimic hydroceles and vice versa. Excision takes place under a short general anaesthetic but be cautious intervening in young patients, due to the possibility of causing an obstruction to the spermatic tubules. If fertility is important then counsel waiting until the patient's family is complete.

Varicoceles are common and are a source of controversy. There is a higher incidence of varicocele in sub-fertile men, and repairing the varicocele has been shown to improve semen analyses and more recently improve live pregnancy rates. The mechanism for impacting normal testicular development is venous stasis in dilated veins which affect the temperature that the testis is exposed to as well as increased exposure to toxic metabolites. Repair can be done via an embolisation approach (involving interventional radiology), open (retroperitoneal, inguinal, sub-inguinal) or laparoscopic approaches. Enquire about fertility and successful pregnancies, how much the varicocele is impacting quality of life and if there is a size discrepancy between testes.

TOP TIP:

Young patients with a larger varicocele and a small testis may well benefit from repair. The middle-aged man with normal testis, a completed family and an incidental diagnosis of a varicocele on an US performed for scrotal pain probably doesn't.

All scrotal surgery carries risks; therefore, ensure that the patient is furnished with a detailed patient information leaflet. The authors quote at least a 10% risk of haematoma for all scrotal surgery as well as a small risk of damage to the vas/vessels. We would also suggest that no matter how confident you are of the clinical diagnosis, a pre-operative US testes is advisable.

THE CLINIC

4.3 HAEMATURIA

There are clear local and national guidelines on when to refer in a patient on an urgent basis for investigations, and most departments run a haematuria clinic which enables rapid access to appropriate diagnostics for these patients. The causes of haematuria are numerous but the common causes you will see include: urological tumours, infections, trauma and stones. There is an important divide between visible (VH) and non-visible (nVH) haematuria. The patient with VH has a 20% risk of an underlying urological malignancy and requires a history, examination (including a DRE or VE), urine culture, blood tests (including GFR, FBC and a PSA for male patients), upper tract imaging (CT urogram) and a flexible cystoscopy. The patient with nVH has a much lower risk of sinister pathology (5%) but requires the same investigations, albeit with US KUB instead of CT urography. Some departments send urine for cytology.

Key points in the history include:
- Duration of symptoms
- Painful or painless
- History of being a smoker, chemical exposure
- Family history of urological malignancy
- Past medical history of urological malignancy
- history of anticoagulants.

If the above investigations are all normal then reassurance can be provided, along with instructions to return if further bleeding occurs. Persistent nVH may be a marker for subsequent renal disease, so such patients should be asked to see a renal physician.

THE CLINIC

4.4 RAISED PSA

This is a common referral and, due to the concern of an underlying prostate cancer, often results in an urgent (two-week rule) referral. There are local and national age-specific PSA values, with the current UK NICE threshold of below 3.0 for a man aged 50–69. Over the last 5–10 years there has been a shift in how this should be managed, with most centres now offering an upfront multi-parametric MRI. This should be reported using a standardised scheme called PIRADS, which gives a grading as to the chance of significant prostate cancer being present (graded 1–5). The MRI characteristics will then guide the urologist on how best to proceed and also how best to biopsy the prostate.

Key points from the history include:
- Age and ethnicity of the patient
- History of urinary tract infection
- Family history of prostate cancer
- Any problems with erections or continence
- Any symptoms of back pain, weight loss or lower limb neurology.

Even with a pre-visit MRI, the authors still maintain that a DRE is important. Check a urine dipstick (and send it for culture if considering a biopsy) and ask about anticoagulants.

THE CLINIC

4.5 MALE LOWER URINARY TRACT SYMPTOMS

This is another huge topic – the assessment and management of the patient with LUTS takes time to learn but it is one of the most common referrals to urology.

Key points to consider when on-call are:
- Is there any risk to the upper tracts?
- Is there an underlying malignancy?
- How much are the symptoms affecting quality of life?
- Is the patient suitable for an intervention?

The history should cover most of the above points – also, remember to ask about any "red-flag" symptoms. Teasing out what symptoms or symptom the patient has that are causing concern is really important. A urine dip and a full abdominal, genital and rectal examination are mandatory. Check renal function and a PSA. A flow rate, post-void residual and a frequency–volume chart are useful screening tools. Broadly speaking, the management options comprise: conservative approaches (lifestyle changes), medical treatments (alpha-blocker, 5 alpha-reductase inhibitor or an anticholinergic) and then surgery. Established procedures include trans-urethral resection of the prostate and laser prostatectomy (greenlight or holmium laser enucleation). Recently, there has been an increase in operative options available to manage benign prostatic hyperplasia and this field is likely to continue to develop. Newer interventions include some minimally invasive treatments, such as prostatic urethral lifts or steam treatment.

TOP TIP:

The **red-flag symptoms** are: haematuria, recurrent infections, back pain and leg weakness.

THE CLINIC

CHAPTER 5: THE OPERATING THEATRE

5.1 CLASSIFICATION OF EMERGENCY SURGERY

The **National Confidential Enquiry into Patient Outcome and Death** (NCEPOD) is an independent organisation and registered charity in the UK. It reports on clinical practice and potential remediable factors in the peri-operative course of the surgical patient. The very first report was commissioned in 1995 under a different name; now it reports on yearly data and makes recommendations on how to improve patient care.

Key points highlighted in the past include that over 80% of peri-operative deaths (defined as occurring less than 30 days after the operation date) occur in emergency operations. Often, a patient's comorbid status is not fully understood in the emergency scenario, and reversible impairments are not reversed pre-operatively (i.e. patients are not optimised before surgery). This is often a careful balancing act within the time pressures that most emergencies present. NCEPOD also suggests sensible time frames to operate in. Ideally, only life- and limb-threatening cases should take place after midnight. In urology therefore, we endeavour to perform our emergency cases within working hours. The exceptions to that rule include acute testicular torsions, infected obstructed systems and trauma cases, which can present at any time and require prompt intervention.

Classification	Description	Time to theatre
IMMEDIATE	Immediate life-saving, or limb or organ-saving intervention. Resuscitation will occur simultaneous with surgical treatment.	Minutes
URGENT	Acute onset or deterioration of condition that threatens life, limb or organ survival.	Hours
EXPEDITED	Stable patient requiring early intervention for a condition not threatening life, limb or organ.	Days
ELECTIVE	Surgical procedure planned or booked in advance of routine admission to hospital.	Planned procedure (weeks/months)

Table 5.1: NCEPOD classification of emergency surgery

When booking a patient onto an emergency list, you will usually be asked to classify the operation and it is important that you classify cases accordingly. Suspected testicular torsion, whilst not a life- or limb-threatening case, should be classified as "immediate" in order to have the best chance of saving the testicle.

NCEPOD is a UK phenomenon but the principles of emergency operating apply to healthcare institutions worldwide.

THE OPERATING THEATRE

5.2 THE WHO SURGICAL SAFETY CHECKLIST

The WHO checklist has now been globally implemented to help reduce errors and adverse events in the operating theatre. The exact content of the checklist is variable upon local practice and the official protocol will typically be displayed on the walls in all operating theatres. It has now become commonplace to carry out the checklist at 3 key stages of the procedure:

'SIGN IN'

Prior to induction of anaesthesia, with a nurse and anaesthetist:

- Patient confirms identity, procedure and consent
- The operative site marking is confirmed (if applicable)
- Imaging relevant to the patient is available and/or displayed
- Any allergies are noted
- Anaesthetic equipment, medications and other monitoring equipment is checked
- The anaesthetist will note a potentially difficult airway
- Any risk of significant blood loss is noted and pre-emptive measures taken.

'TIME OUT'

After the patient is anaesthetised, prior to skin incision:

- All team members introduced themselves by name and role
- The patients identity is confirmed along with the procedure
- Antibiotic prophylaxis is requested if required
- The surgical, anaesthetic or nursing team can report any anticipated critical events.

'SIGN OUT'

After the procedure, prior to the patient leaving the operating room:

- The nursing staff and surgical team confirm the exact procedure performed
- Instrument, needle and swab counts should be correct
- Specimens should be labelled appropriately
- Any equipment problems should be noted and addressed
- Key concerns for recovery and ongoing management should be expressed.

It is important to be familiar with these protocols in your local department as it is paramount to follow them to ensure patient safety. Furthermore, you may be asked to play an important role in conducting any of the above safety checks.

THE OPERATING THEATRE

5.3 PLACING A PATIENT ON THE EMERGENCY LIST

Once the decision has been made to take a patient to theatre, there are several steps you need to carry out to facilitate this to ensure that the patient is ready.

1. Make sure the patient is informed about the procedure. They will need consenting and marking for their procedure. If you are not happy with taking consent, make sure your senior is doing this.

2. Fill out the necessary paperwork (paper or electronic, depending on your hospital) to book the patient onto the emergency list. Often you will need to make clear where the patient is (for example, in the emergency department or in a particular ward), what specialist equipment you might need (e.g. image intensifier), who will be performing the operation and how to contact them.

3. Inform the theatre coordinator either face-to-face or over the phone.

4. Inform the on-call anaesthetist. They will want to know what comorbidities the patient has, their exercise function, allergies, and recent blood tests and other important investigations, so have these to hand when talking to them.

5. Think carefully about who else needs to know that this patient is going to theatre. For example, if an image intensifier is needed to place a ureteric stent for a patient, you also need to inform the on-call radiographer. Sometimes the theatre coordinator will do this for you, but you need to check.

6. It is important to ask what else is on the emergency operating list and when you might be able to operate on your patient. There may be a queue of patients and if you feel your case should take clinical priority, you will need to negotiate this with the other teams waiting to operate. If you are not the operating surgeon, it is best to defer to them for this.

If there is a delay, you may want to utilise your time well by seeing other patients, for example. However, it is sensible that you keep an eye on the time and regularly check in with theatres for an update of when you might be able to start your case.

5.4 CONSENT AND MARKING

You will need to make sure the patient is informed of the treatment decision and that they have consented for the operation. It is important to mark where the site of the procedure will be (i.e. if this is an exploration of the left testicle, make sure you have drawn an arrow on the left side of the patient).

Consent should ideally be taken by the operating surgeon. You will need to consult your local hospital's guidance to select the appropriate consent form, but in principle, in the UK, it involves completing a consent form 1, 2, 3 or 4:

- *Consent form 1* is for procedures under regional or general anaesthetic where an adult patient has capacity to consent
- *Consent form 2* is for paediatric patients
- *Consent form 3* is for procedures where the patient is fully conscious, under local anaesthetic (e.g. flexible cystoscopic guided catheter insertion)
- *Consent form 4* is for procedures where the patient lacks capacity to consent (e.g. dementia); if you are signing this, it is advisable to make sure your senior also countersigns.

In the UK, there are many different leaflets that are commonly used to provide patients with information prior to an operation. It is considered best practice in the UK to use information leaflets from the British Association of Urology Surgeons (BAUS) website (www.baus.org.uk), which can be accessed, printed and given to the patient. Make sure you have given a copy to the patient and asked them to read it before the operation. For elective operations, best practice states that patients should receive these information leaflets in clinic, and on the day of surgery you must check they have read and understood the operation, its risks and alternatives before confirming they have given their informed consent. This is not always practical in the emergency setting.

THE OPERATING THEATRE

5.5 PREPARING A PATIENT FOR THEATRE

Inform the nurse looking after the patient, and the nurse in charge of the ward, that the patient is going to theatre. They will need to make sure that:

- The patient is dressed in a gown
- The patient is wearing thromboembolic deterrent (TED) stockings (make sure you have prescribed these)
- The patient is kept NBM, including stopping any NG feed; you should also tell the patient directly not to eat or drink
- The pre-operative checklists are completed on the ward in line with individual hospital policy; often, the patient will not be able to leave the ward until all the necessary paperwork is completed and available, so save time and make sure this is being sorted as soon as possible
- Any pre-meds the anaesthetist may have requested (e.g. PPI) are given to the patient appropriately.

Make sure that you have personally checked all the patient's blood results: check the clotting screen is normal (INR is within normal range if the patient is on warfarin), haemoglobin levels are normal (or transfuse pre-op if required), platelet levels are normal (or transfuse pre-op if required) and serum potassium is normal (high or low values are an issue during an anaesthetic and need to be corrected as soon as possible).

TOP TIP:

Make sure that you check the drug chart:

- Check if the patient has had any anticoagulants recently (most surgeons will operate with a patient on aspirin, but clopidogrel, warfarin and the newer direct thrombin inhibitors must be stopped)
- Check with the anaesthetist, but as a general rule, patients should take all their regular medication with a small sip of water (particularly Parkinson's medication, antihypertensives, etc.).

THE OPERATING THEATRE

5.6 BENEFITS AND RISKS OF SPECIFIC SURGICAL PROCEDURES

The following section details information typically included on the consent form for the commonest urology procedures you might encounter when on-call. The lists are not exhaustive and serve as a guide only. The risks and benefits of surgery should be discussed using language and terms that the patient can fully understand. It is important to tailor each consent process to the individual patient.

5.6.1 FLEXIBLE CYSTOSCOPY

BENEFITS OF THE OPERATION:
- Diagnostic procedure to examine the inside of the bladder
- Assist with difficult catheter insertion

POSSIBLE RISKS:
- Urinary tract infection
- Dysuria
- Bleeding
- Urinary retention

5.6.2 RIGID CYSTOSCOPY +/- BLADDER BIOPSY

BENEFITS OF THE OPERATION:
- Diagnostic procedure to examine the inside of the bladder
- Diagnose suspected bladder cancer

POSSIBLE RISKS:
- Urinary tract infection
- Dysuria
- Bleeding
- Urinary retention
- Bladder perforation
- Temporary insertion of urinary catheter

THE OPERATING THEATRE

5.6.3 CIRCUMCISION

BENEFITS OF THE OPERATION:

- Treat phimosis and restore function

POSSIBLE RISKS:

- Swelling of the penis
- Increased sensitivity of the glans which can last for up to two weeks
- Permanent altered or reduced sensation in the glans
- Infection of the incision, requiring antibiotics or surgical drainage
- Bleeding from the wound, occasionally requiring a further procedure
- Dissatisfaction with the cosmetic result

5.6.4 HYDROCELE REPAIR

BENEFITS OF THE OPERATION:

- Treat pain and/or altered cosmesis

POSSIBLE RISKS:

- Swelling, discomfort and bruising of the scrotum lasting several days
- Haematoma around the testicle which resolves slowly or needs surgical drainage
- Infection in the incision or testicle, requiring antibiotics or surgical drainage
- Recurrence of the hydrocele
- Chronic scrotal pain

THE OPERATING THEATRE

5.6.5 SCROTAL EXPLORATION FOR SUSPECTED TESTICULAR TORSION

BENEFITS OF THE OPERATION:

- Treat testicular torsion and prevent permanent damage or loss of the testicle

POSSIBLE RISKS:

- If torsion of the testis is confirmed, the need to fix both testicles in the scrotum immediately
- Swelling, discomfort and bruising of the scrotum lasting several days
- Need to remove the affected testicle if it is too damaged to recover
- Palpable fixation stitches through the scrotal skin
- Haematoma around the testicle which resolves slowly or needs surgical drainage
- Infection in the incision or testicle, requiring antibiotics or surgical drainage
- Late atrophy of the testicle
- Reduced fertility due to testicular damage caused by temporary interruption of its blood supply

THE OPERATING THEATRE

5.6.6 URETERIC STENT INSERTION

BENEFITS OF THE OPERATION:

- To relieve obstruction to the kidney

POSSIBLE RISKS:

- Mild burning or bleeding on passing urine which can continue until the stent is removed
- Temporary insertion of a catheter, which may cause pain, frequency and bleeding
- A further procedure is required to remove the stent at a later date
- Urinary tract infection
- Failure to get the stent into the ureter, requiring an alternative procedure

5.6.7 SUPRAPUBIC CATHETER INSERTION

BENEFITS OF THE OPERATION:

- To relieve bladder outflow obstruction

POSSIBLE RISKS:

- Mild burning or bleeding on passing urine, lasting for a few days
- Recurrent urinary tract infection, requiring antibiotics
- Blockage of the catheter by debris or blood clots, requiring irrigation and unblocking
- Bladder spasms or bladder pain
- Bladder stone formation
- Inadvertent damage to adjacent structures (e.g. bowel, blood vessels), requiring further surgery

THE OPERATING THEATRE

5.7 WHAT TO ASK YOUR SCRUB NURSE FOR

At the time of booking the case, it is essential that you check with the scrub team that they have the correct equipment needed to perform the operation required. Often your scrub team will not be urology trained and therefore will not automatically know you need X-ray guidance to perform a ureteric stent insertion.

Below is the typically required equipment used for the common operations you would be booking on an emergency list as the urology on-call doctor.

SCROTAL EXPLORATION

Minors set (which typically includes a toothed and non-toothed forceps, a needle holder, stitch scissors and dissecting scissors), diathermy (depending on surgeon choice, both monopolar and bipolar can be used), non-absorbable sutures for the potential orchidopexy, absorbable suture for closure of the dartos muscle, absorbable suture for skin closure and a scrotal support to place on the patient after closing

SCROTAL ABSCESS DRAINAGE

Minors set, diathermy (depending on surgeon choice, both monopolar and bipolar can be used), absorbable suture for closure of dartos, absorbable suture for skin closure, corrugated drain and scrotal support to place on the patient after closing

FLEXIBLE CYSTOSCOPY +/- CATHETER INSERTION

Flexible cystoscope, video stack system, guidewire and open-ended catheter

URETERIC STENT INSERTION

X-ray image intensifier (and radiographer), guidewire (ideally one with a hydrophilic tip), ureteric catheter, contrast, ureteric stent (usually 6Fr, 22–26cm in length, depending on patient size), rigid cystoscope, video stack system and lithotomy leg supports

THE OPERATING THEATRE

CHAPTER 6: PRACTICAL PROCEDURES

6.1 VENEPUNCTURE, IV CANNULATION, TAKING BLOOD CULTURES AND ARTERIAL BLOOD GASES

VENEPUNCTURE

Venepuncture is a core skill which you will have had to demonstrate competency at prior to passing your final examinations at medical school. Below are the basic steps to act as a reminder.

You will need: gloves, needle, vacuum sealed blood collection device, tourniquet, cleaning wipe, dressing, blood bottles, sharps bin.

1. Wash/alcohol gel your hands.
2. Introduce yourself to the patient, check you have the correct, intended patient and gain verbal consent for the procedure.
3. Apply a tourniquet to the patient's arm and palpate a suitable vein.
4. Clean the area with a cleaning wipe.
5. Put on non-sterile gloves.
6. Assemble the needle and blood collection device together and insert the needle into the patient's vein at a 45° angle.
7. Push the required blood bottles onto the blood collection device end and fill to the desired level.
8. Remove the tourniquet then remove the needle from the vein.
9. Cover the puncture mark with a dressing and ask the patient to apply pressure using their other hand.
10. Dispose of your sharps in the sharps bin and the remaining contents of your tray in the appropriate clinical waste bins.
11. Remove your gloves and wash/alcohol gel your hands.
12. Label the bottles correctly, fill out the request card correctly and ensure you place the samples in the correct place for their collection to be sent to the lab (it is usually sensible to confirm this with one of the nursing staff).

Blood bottle top colour	Common blood test requests in urology
Yellow	U&E, bone profile, serum calcium, serum urate/uric acid, serum bicarbonate, PSA
Purple	FBC
Blue	Coagulation screen, INR
Pink	Group and save, cross match

Table 6.1: Blood bottles

It is important to note that the colours can vary between different hospital trusts – this is just a guide. It is sensible to double check with colleagues, the nursing staff or the lab itself that you are using the correct bottle for the test you intend to request, before taking blood from the patient.

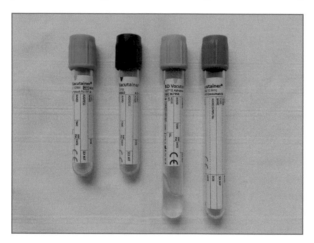

Figure 6.1: Blood bottles

INTRAVENOUS CANNULATION

Intravenous cannulation is a core skill which you will have learnt at medical school. Below are the basic steps to act as a reminder.

You will need: gloves, cannula, tourniquet, dressing, 5ml syringe, 5ml of normal saline, cleaning wipe, sharps bin.

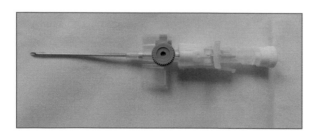

Figure 6.2: Cannula

PROCEDURES

1. Wash/alcohol gel your hands.
2. Introduce yourself and check you have the correct patient. Gain verbal consent for the procedure.
3. Apply a tourniquet to the patient's arm and palpate a suitable vein.
4. Clean the area with a cleaning wipe.
5. Put on non-sterile gloves.
6. Position the cannula and insert the needle into the patient's vein at a 45° angle. Once you see a "*flash-back*", pull the needle back into the cannula and advance it into the vein.
7. Remove the tourniquet then remove the needle from the vein.
8. Place a stopper on the end of the cannula and secure it into place with a dressing.
9. Flush the cannula with 5ml of normal saline.
10. Dispose of your sharps in the sharps bin and the remaining contents of your tray in the appropriate clinical waste bins.
11. Remove your gloves and wash/alcohol gel your hands.
12. Complete your trust proforma for cannula insertion, ensuring you put the correct date and time on the form. This will ensure cannulas are removed before they become an infection risk.

TAKING BLOOD CULTURES

Taking blood cultures is another core skill which you will have learnt at medical school. Below are the basic steps to act as a reminder.

You will need: gloves, needle, vacuum sealed blood collection device, tourniquet, three cleaning wipes, blood culture bottles, sharps bin.

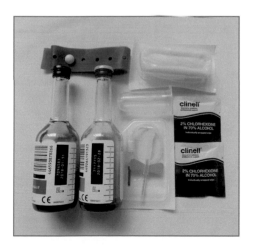

Figure 6.3: Blood culture bottles and equipment

PROCEDURES

1. Wash/alcohol gel your hands.
2. Introduce yourself to the patient, check you have the correct, intended patient and gain verbal consent for the procedure.
3. Apply a tourniquet to the patient's arm and palpate a suitable vein.
4. Clean the area with a cleaning wipe.
5. Put on non-sterile gloves.
6. Assemble the blood culture bottles, remove the caps and swipe the top of each with a clean wipe.
7. Assemble the needle and blood collection device together and insert the needle into the patient's vein at a 45° angle.
8. Push the blood bottles onto the blood collection device end and fill to the desired level. You will need to fill with a minimum of 5ml.
9. Remove the tourniquet then remove the needle from the vein.
10. Cover the puncture mark with a dressing and ask the patient to apply pressure using their other hand.
11. Dispose of your sharps in the sharps bin and the remaining contents of your tray in the appropriate clinical waste bins.
12. Remove your gloves and wash/alcohol gel your hands.
13. Label the bottles correctly, fill out the request card correctly and ensure you place the samples in the correct place for their collection to be sent to the lab (it is usually sensible to confirm this with one of the nursing staff).

TAKING AN ARTERIAL BLOOD GAS

Taking an arterial blood gas (ABG) is another skill which you will have learnt at medical school. Below are the basic steps to act as a reminder.

You will need: needle, blood gas syringe, cleaning wipe, dressing, sharps bin.

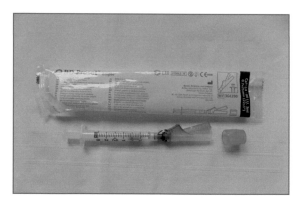

Figure 6.4: ABG syringe

PROCEDURES

1. Wash/alcohol gel your hands.
2. Introduce yourself to the patient, check you have the correct, intended patient and gain verbal consent for the procedure.
3. Palpate the radial artery at the patient's wrist.
4. Clean the area with a cleaning wipe.
5. Put on non-sterile gloves.
6. Assemble the blood gas syringe and needle; insert the needle into the patient's radial artery at a 90° angle.
7. The syringe should fill by itself due to the patient's blood pressure (if you are in the right place!).
8. Cover the puncture mark with a dressing and ask the patient to apply pressure using their other hand.
9. Dispose of your sharps in the sharps bin and the remaining contents of your tray in the appropriate clinical waste bins.
10. Remove your gloves and wash/alcohol gel your hands.
11. Move quickly to your nearest blood gas machine to run the sample as soon as possible.

PROCEDURES

6.2 URINE ANALYSIS

PERFORMING A URINE DIPSTICK

Dipstick testing a urine sample is a skill you will have demonstrated before. Many hospitals have automated machines that will read the dipstick test for you. Alternatively, you can read the dipstick yourself, using the colour guide on the container. Below are the basic steps to act as a reminder.

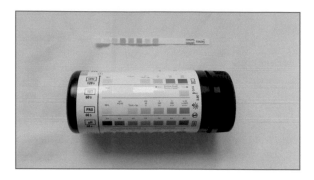

Figure 6.5: Urine dipstick

1. Ask the patient to perform a urine sample in a clean white-topped container.
2. Wash/alcohol gel your hands and put on gloves.
3. Remove a dipstick and submerge the entire strip in the urine sample.
4. You can either:
   a. Place it in the automated machine with the strip side facing up and follow the instructions on the machine

   OR

   b. Carefully shake off the excess urine from the strip and place it down to develop for one minute.
5. Interpret the test by holding it next to the sticker on the side of the test strip bottle and use the colour indicators to determine your result.
6. Record this in the patient's notes, along with the time and date.

OBTAINING A MID-STREAM URINE SAMPLE (MSU)

Patients usually perform this themselves, but you must carefully instruct the patient on how to perform it correctly. Otherwise, there is a significant risk of contamination and false readings. The patient must use a sterile

PROCEDURES

(usually white-topped) specimen container provided by the hospital. In male patients, the foreskin (if it is present) should ideally be retracted; in female patients, the labia must be parted to avoid specimen contamination. Ask the patient to:

1) Begin voiding
2) Collect the specimen mid-flow
3) Secure the container
4) Present it to you for testing using the urine dipstick as above. It can also be sent for microscopy if required.

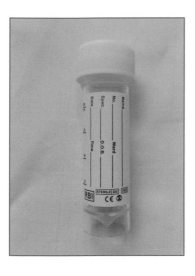

Figure 6.6: Sterile sample pot

CATHETER SPECIMEN OF URINE (CSU)

This sample is taken directly from the patient's catheter and not from the bag. It will usually involve blocking the patient's catheter for 10–15 minutes prior to collecting the specimen.

βHCG URINE TEST

This is a pregnancy test that can be performed on a urine sample obtained using the method above. It is often performed at the same time as a urine dipstick test. Manufacturer instructions will vary, so it is important to read the instructions for the specific test you are using. Some hospitals have automated machines to perform this test. In principle, you will need to cover the active strip of the βHCG test in the patient's urine, either by dipping it directly into the specimen pot or using the pipette provided to cover the active strip in urine. Leave the test to develop for 1–3 minutes, depending

PROCEDURES

on the manufacturer's instructions, and record the results in the patient's notes with the date and time.

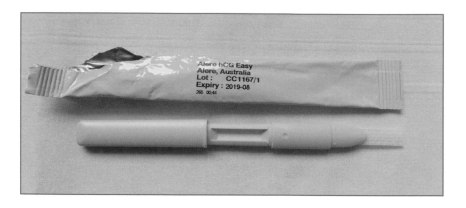

Figure 6.7: βHCG test

6.3 URETHRAL CATHETERISATION

This is a fundamental skill in urology and as you get more experienced, you will no doubt be asked to help place difficult catheters. Below are the basic steps to act as a reminder.

What you need: catheter pack, cleaning solution, two tubes of lubricating gel (containing local anaesthetic), catheter (check it has a 10ml pre-filled syringe of sterile water for injecting the balloon: if it doesn't, you will need a 10ml syringe and 10ml of sterile water) and a catheter bag.

1. Wash/alcohol gel your hands.
2. Introduce yourself to the patient and check you have the correct patient. Explain what you will be doing and gain verbal consent for the procedure.
3. Prepare a catheter trolley and ensure, in a sterile way, that you have the above items.
4. Expose the patient and then wash/alcohol gel your hands and put on sterile gloves.
5. Retract the foreskin, if present, and clean the glans penis.
6. Pass two tubes of lubricating gel gently down the urethra. It is sensible to inject these slowly to avoid stretching the urethra with a sudden injection of a large volume of gel, which is more painful for patients. Make the patient aware this will sting.
7. Pass the catheter all the way down the urethra, until the hilt of the catheter is at the end of the urethra, thus ensuring the balloon is well past the bladder neck.
8. Inflate the balloon with 10ml of sterile water. The volume required to inflate a catheter balloon is always written on the packaging, so confirm the volume before you proceed.
9. Attach the catheter bag.
10. Ensure the foreskin (if present) is retracted back over the glans of the penis.
11. Tidy up all your disposables into the yellow waste bag in the catheter pack, remove your gloves and wash your hands.
12. Record your activity in the patient's notes with the date and time.
13. Go back to check the residual volume drained from the catheter (as sufficient time should have passed now to record a true residual volume) and record this in the patient's notes.

PROCEDURES

If inserting a 3-way urethral catheter, your indication would be for visible haematuria and clot retention. You can follow the above steps exactly; however, be mindful that these catheters require more fluid (commonly 30ml) to fill the balloon. (Again, confirm this by checking the packaging.) Once you have inserted a 3-way catheter, you will need to washout the bladder with a bladder syringe and normal saline or sterile water until all the clots are removed and the urine is clearer. Then you should attach irrigation to the third channel. Again, be sure you have attached the catheter bag and irrigation tubing to the correct channel (see 'Instruments in urology' section).

PROCEDURES

6.4 SUPRAPUBIC CATHETERISATION

This procedure can be associated with significant morbidity and even mortality. What follows is a guide, but unless you are familiar with suprapubic catheters, it is sensible you enlist senior support for this procedure.

Suprapubic catheters should be inserted under direct vision and/or ultrasound guidance to minimise bowel injury. They can be used in certain emergency situations provided that 1) the patient is slim enough, 2) you can confidently feel their bladder well above the pubic symphysis and 3) they have no history of previous lower abdominal surgery. Again, it is sensible to discuss all of this with your senior and only proceed with their supervision.

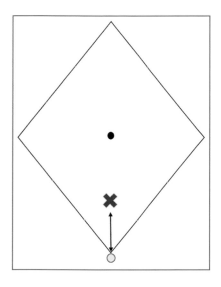

Figure 6.8: Diagram of the ideal location to insert a suprapubic catheter: two finger-breadths above the pubic symphysis (yellow dot), red X marks the spot

There are different suprapubic catheter insertion kits and no real evidence exists that one is better or safer than the other. The following is a description of the commonly used Seldinger principle for inserting a suprapubic catheter.

What you need: catheter pack, cleaning solution such as aqueous betadine, one tube of lubricating gel (containing local anaesthetic), suprapubic catheter pack (suprapubic catheter, guidewire, two 10ml syringes, dilating trocar, small blade, large white needle), catheter bag and 10ml 1% lignocaine.

1. Wash/alcohol gel your hands.
2. Introduce yourself to the patient and check you have the correct patient. Explain what you intend to do and gain verbal consent for the procedure.

PROCEDURES

3. Ensure you inspect the abdomen: check that you can easily feel a palpable bladder several finger widths above the symphysis pubis and that there are no lower abdominal scars.

4. Prepare a catheter trolley and ensure you have the items listed above laid out on the trolley in a sterile way.

5. Put on sterile gloves and prepare your tray.

6. Draw up the lignocaine into one of the 10ml syringes and mount an orange needle on it. Draw up 10ml of sterile water in the other syringe.

7. Expose the patient and then wash/alcohol gel your hands and put on sterile gloves.

8. Clean the suprapubic area with aqueous betadine.

9. Palpate two finger breadths above the symphysis pubis – this is where you will insert the catheter. Inject the local anaesthetic first under the skin (using an orange needle) and then deeper down the tract using the white needle.

10. Next, begin to withdraw on the now-empty syringe. Once you aspirate urine you know you are in the bladder. Now you can remove the syringe, but leave the needle in place.

11. Pass the guidewire down the needle into the bladder and remove the needle, leaving the guidewire in place.

12. Next, make a skin incision around the wire to allow you to pass the dilator and catheter. (It is sensible to cut slightly deeper, down to the rectus sheath, so as to make it easier to pass the dilator and catheter.)

13. Now pass the dilator down over the guidewire and into the bladder. You will need to use quite a bit of force, and you need to be sure that the outer sheath is in the bladder, so push it in further than you think.

14. Then remove the inside of the dilating trocar with the guidewire; you should get a flush back of urine at this point.

15. Quickly pass the catheter in through the outer dilating sheath before the bladder empties, and inflate the balloon with 10ml of sterile water.

16. Attach the catheter bag.

17. Remove the outer dilating sheath by pulling on the tab to divide it.

18. Tidy up all your disposables into the appropriate clinical waste bins, place your sharps into the sharps bin, remove your gloves and wash your hands.

19. Record your activity in the patient's notes with the date and time.

20. Go back to check the residual volume drained from the catheter (as sufficient time should have passed now to record a true residual volume) and record this in the patient's notes.

PROCEDURES

6.5 PENILE BLOCK

A penile block need only be performed in an emergency setting, most commonly to help you to reduce a paraphimosis or perform a dorsal slit for phimosis preventing catheterisation. When properly administered, this should ensure the whole penile shaft, glans penis and foreskin are numb.

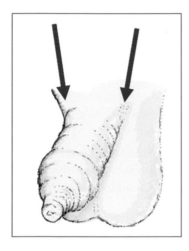

Figure 6.9: Diagram to demonstrate where to inject your penile block (red arrows) either side of the penile suspensory ligament, which lies in the midline

You will need: non-sterile gloves, alcohol wipe for the skin, 20ml 1% lignocaine (plain), a large bore drawing up needle, a 20ml syringe, a narrower gauged needle for administering the block (i.e. 23G blue needle).

1. Wash/alcohol gel your hands.
2. Introduce yourself to the patient and check you have the correct patient. Gain verbal consent for the procedure.
3. Draw up 20ml 1% lignocaine (plain) and check the patient has no allergies.
4. Clean the dorsal aspect of the base of the penis, and the ventral aspect of the peno-scrotal junction with an alcohol wipe.
5. Palpate the suspensory ligament of the penis in the midline coming off the pubic symphysis. Inject either side of that ligament to anaesthetise the nerve bundle running laterally in the penile shaft.
6. Inject also at the peno-scrotal junction on the ventral aspect of the penis to catch the nerves supplying the frenulum.
7. Wait a few minutes for the block to take effect and test it before performing any procedure.
8. Don't forget to record this in the patient's notes with the date and time.

PROCEDURES

6.6 REDUCTION OF A PARAPHIMOSIS

This is a two-handed technique. You can attempt it without using a penile block if the patient permits.

You will need: gloves and lubricating gel (containing local anaesthetic).

1. Wash/alcohol gel your hands.
2. Introduce yourself to the patient and check you have the correct patient. Gain verbal consent for the procedure.
3. Put on non-sterile gloves.
4. Cover the end of the penis with lubricating gel (containing local anaesthetic).
5. Place your index and middle fingers on either side behind the retracted, swollen foreskin and your thumbs on the tip of the glans penis.
6. Simultaneously push down with your thumbs and pull forward with your fingers to bring the foreskin back over the glans penis. Sometimes a period of compression of the oedematous glans and foreskin prior to the reduction manoeuvre is required.

This is usually successful, but occasionally patients don't present for some time and have such significant swelling that they require a dorsal slit or circumcision under local anaesthetic, which is best done in theatre. Contact your senior in this situation.

PROCEDURES

AUTHOR BIOGRAPHIES

Mr Andrew Chetwood, **BMedSci (Hons), MBChB (Hons), FRCS (Urol)**, is a consultant urologist at Frimley Health NHS Foundation Trust. He has a wide-ranging general urological practice with a special interest in reconstructive urology.

Mr Hamid Abboudi, **BSc, MBBS, PG CERT HBE, FRCS (Urol)**, is a urology consultant at Imperial College Healthcare NHS Trust specialising in endourology. He has a particular interest in the medical and surgical management of patients with kidney stones and benign prostate diseases.

Miss Charlotte Dunford, **MBBS, BSc (Hons), FRCS (Urol)**, is a consultant urologist at the Norfolk and Norwich University Hospitals NHS Trust. She has a sub-specialist interest in adolescent, functional and reconstructive urology.

INDEX

ABCDE approach   37, 57, 59
Abdominal aortic aneurysm   26, 28, 32, 64
Abdominal drain   55
Amoxicillin   15, 43
Analgesia   13, 27, 39, 40, 45, 58, 60
Anti-emetics   14
Antibiotics   14–15, 29, 31, 39, 43, 45, 58, 59, 60
Anticoagulation   5, 26, 30, 47, 54, 64, 67, 68, 76
Arterial blood gas   86–7
Aspirin   54, 76

Bacteriuria, asymptomatic   42–3
Beta-HCG (βHCG)   8, 89–90
Bladder biopsy   77
Bladder syringe   18, 92
Bladder washout   18, 30, 35, 56, 59
Blood cultures   85–6
Blood glucose   51–3
Blood tests   8, 9, 26, 29, 30, 33, 67, 74, 84
Blood transfusion   6–7

Catheter bag   17, 18, 19–20, 91, 93
Catheter guide   16
Catheter specimen of urine   89
Catheter, blocked   5, 35
Catheter, difficult   22, 34–5, 77, 91
Catheter, dislodged   5, 35
Catheter, suprapubic   18, 34, 35, 80, 93–4
Catheter, 3-way   16–17, 30, 35, 56, 60, 92
Catheter, 2-way   16–17, 18, 56
Cefuroxime   15
Circumcision   36, 60, 78, 96
Clopidogrel   54, 76
Clot retention   30, 92
Co-amoxiclav   15
Consent   7, 29, 73, 74, 75, 77
CT KUB   8, 12, 26, 42, 64
CT urography   8, 11, 12, 30, 44, 67

Cystectomy   7, 55, 60
Cystogram   11, 38
Cystoscope, flexible   21, 34, 35, 77, 81
Cystoscope, rigid   22, 23, 77, 81

Diabetic patients   5, 51, 52–3
Dipyridamole   54
Diuresis   33, 48, 50
DMSA   12

Electrolyte requirements   48
Epididymal cyst   60, 65–6
Epididymo-orchitis   29, 45
Fluid maintenance   48–9

Gentamicin   15
Guidewire   3, 21, 22, 23, 34, 35, 81, 93, 94

Haematuria   8, 16, 26, 30, 38, 56, 67, 69
Hydrocele   45, 60, 65–6, 78
Hydronephrosis   12, 33, 42–3
Hyperglycaemia   52
Hypoglycaemia   51, 58

Instillagel   19
Intravenous fluids   33, 48–9, 50
IVU   11, 26, 38

KUB, X-ray   11, 27, 64

Lower urinary tract symptoms   69

MAG3   12
Marking   29, 73, 74, 75
Medical expulsive therapy   27
Metronidazole   15
Mid-stream urine   6, 88–9
MRI   12, 68
Multidisciplinary team (MDT)   7

NCEPOD   71–2
Nephrectomy   6–7, 38, 60

Nephrostomy   3, 26, 42–3, 55
Nitrofurantoin   15, 43

Paraphimosis   36, 45, 95
Penile amputation   39
Penile block   36, 40, 60, 95, 96
Percutaneous nephrolithotomy   7, 55, 64
Phimosis   34, 36, 45, 78, 95
PIRADS   68
Post-obstructive diuresis   33, 48, 50
Pregnancy   26, 42–3, 66, 89
Priapism   40–1
Prostatectomy   7, 55, 60–1, 69
PSA   9, 30, 67, 68, 69, 84

Referrals   4–5
Renal colic   8, 26–7
Renal stones   11, 12, 26–7, 64
Rivaroxaban   54

Scrotal abscess   60, 81
Scrotal exploration   60, 79, 81
Scrotal swelling   45, 65–6
Sensor™ wire   23
Septic patient   31, 43, 51
Shock   48, 57, 58
Stents   3, 11, 22, 23, 26, 42, 54, 55, 74, 80, 81

TED stockings   76
Testicular torsion   29, 45, 60, 71, 72, 79
Testicular tumour   7, 28, 29, 65

Ticagrelor   54
Transurethral resection of the prostate   7, 57, 59
Trauma, bladder   11, 38
Trauma, genital   39
Trauma, renal   11, 37–8, 45
Trauma, scrotal   28, 39
Trauma, urethral   11, 17, 38, 56
Trial without catheter (TWOC)   32, 33, 56
Trimethoprim   15, 43
TUR syndrome   59

Ultrasound   12, 60, 93 – see also US KUB
Urethrogram   11, 38
Urinalysis   26, 29, 30, 31
Urinary retention, acute   8, 32
Urinary retention, children   45
Urinary retention, chronic   33
Urinary tract infection   6, 31, 42, 68, 77, 80
Urine dipstick   32, 42, 68, 88, 89
US KUB   8, 12, 43, 64, 67

Varicocele   65–6
Venepuncture   83–4

Ward round   47
Warfarin   54, 76
Water requirement   48
WHO checklist   73
WHO pain ladder   13